Study Guide and Solutions Manual

for

Essentials of Genetics

Eighth Edition

Klug • Cummings • Spencer • Palladino

Harry Nickla

Creighton University

PEARSON

Boston Columbus Indianapolis New York San Francisco Upper Saddle River
Amsterdam Cape Town Dubai London Madrid Milan Munich Paris Montréal Toronto
Delhi Mexico City São Paulo Sydney Hong Kong Seoul Singapore Taipei Tokyo

Editor-in-Chief: Beth Wilbur

Executive Director of Development: Deborah Gale

Senior Acquisitions Editor: Michael Gillespie

Editorial Assistant: Edward Lee

Managing Editor, Production: Mike Early

Production Project Manager and Manufacturing Buyer: Dorothy Cox

Executive Marketing Manager: Lauren Harp

Project Management and Composition: Integra Software Services, Hema Latha

Supplement Cover Design: Seventeenth Street Studios

Main Text Cover Design: Jana Anderson

Cover Photo Credit: Roger Harris/Photo Researchers Inc.

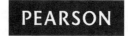

www.pearsonhighered.com

ISBN 10:   0-321-85721-6

ISBN 13: 978-0-321-85721-7

2 3 4 5 6 7 8 9—EBM—16 15 14 13

Contents

How to Increase Your Chances of Success in Genetics:

1. Attend Class
2. Read the Book
3. Do the Assigned Problems
4. Don't Cram
5. Study When There Are No Tests
6. Develop Confidence from Effort
7. Set Disciplined Study Goals
8. Learn Concepts
9. Be Careful with Old Exams
10. Don't "Second Guess" the Teacher

A first course in genetics can be a humbling experience for many students. The intent of this book is to help you understand introductory genetics as presented in the text **Essentials of Genetics** (8th edition). It is possible that the lowest grades received in one's major, or even in one's undergraduate career, may be in genetics. It is not unusual for some students to become frustrated with their own inability to succeed in genetics. This frustration is felt by teachers as they field the following types of student comments:

"I studied all the material but failed your test."

"I must have a mental block to it. I just don't get it. I just don't understand what you are asking."

"Where did you get that question? I didn't see anything like that in the book or in my notes."

"This is the first test I have **ever** failed."

"I helped three of my friends last night and I got the lowest grade."

"I am getting a 'D' in your course and I have never received less than a 'B' in my whole life."

"I stayed up all night studying for your exam and I still failed."

Similar to Algebra

Think back to the first time you encountered "word problems" in your first algebra class. How many times did you ask yourself, your parents, or your teacher the following classic question?

"I hate word problems, I just can't understand them, and why do I need to learn this anyway, I'll never use it?"

At that time, you had two choices: drop out and be afraid of problem solving for the rest of your life (which, unfortunately, happens too often) or regroup, seek help, strip away distractions, and focus on learning something new and powerful. Because you are taking genetics, you probably succeeded in algebra, perhaps with difficulty at first, and you will probably succeed in genetics.

In algebra, you were forced to convert something real and dynamic (e.g., two trains leaving at different times from different stations at different speeds) to a somewhat abstract formula that could be applied to an infinite number of similar problems. In genetics you will again learn something new. It will involve the conversion of something real and dynamic (genes, chromosomes, hereditary elements, gamete formation, gene splicing, and evolution) to an array of general concepts (similar to mathematical formulas) that will allow you to predict the outcome of an infinite number of presently known and yet-to-be-discovered phenomena relating to the origin and maintenance of life.

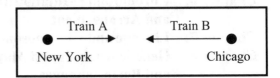

Mental Pictures and Symbols

When working almost any "word" problem, it is often helpful to make a simple drawing that relates, in space, the primary participants. From that drawing, one can often predict or estimate a likely outcome. A mathematical formula and its solution provide the precise outcome. To understand genetics, it is often helpful to make drawings of the participants, whether they be crosses ($Aa \times Aa$), gametes (A or a), or molecules (anticodon interacting with codon).

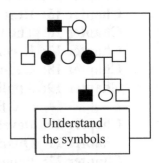

As with algebra, symbols used to represent a multitude of structures, movements, and interactions are abstract, informative, and fundamental to understanding the discipline. It is the set of symbols and their interrelationships that comprise the concepts that make up the framework of genetics. Test questions and problems exemplify the concepts and may be completely unfamiliar to the student; nevertheless, they refer directly to the basic concepts of genetics.

Students: Read All of This Section First!!!

Attendance and Attention Are Mandatory

Many professors do not take attendance in lectures; therefore, it is likely that some students will opt to take a day off now and then. Unless those students are excellent readers and excellent students in general, continual absences will usually result in failure.

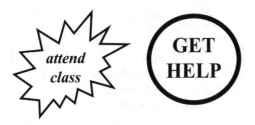

Remember how difficult it was to set up and understand the first algebra word problem on your own? It is likely that your ultimate source of understanding came from the course instructor. While using the text is important in your understanding of genetics, the teacher can walk you through the concepts and strategies much more efficiently than a text because a text is organized in a sequential manner. A good teacher can "cut and paste" an idea from here and there as needed.

To benefit from the wisdom of the instructor, the student must concentrate during the lecture session rather than sit, passively taking notes, assuming that the ideas can be figured out at a later date. Too often the student will not be able to relate to notes passively taken weeks before. In addition, the instructor will not be able to cover all the material in the text. Parts will be emphasized whereas other areas may be omitted entirely.

There is no magic formula for understanding genetics or any other discipline of significance. Learning anything, especially at the college level, requires time, patience, and confidence. First, a student must be willing to focus on the subject matter for an hour or so each day over the entire semester (quarter, trimester, etc.). Study time must be free of distractions and pressured by realistic goals.

The student must be patient and disciplined. It will be necessary to study when there are no assignments due and no tests looming.

Since it is the instructor who writes and grades the tests, who is in a better position to prepare the students for those tests?

The majority of successful students are willing to read the text ahead of the lecture material, spend time thinking about the concepts and examples, and work as many sample problems as possible. They study for a period of time, stop, then return to review the most difficult areas. They do not try to cram information into marathon study sessions a few nights before the examinations. Although some may get away with that practice on occasion, more often than not, understanding the concepts in genetics requires more mature study habits and preparation.

Perhaps a Different Way of Thinking

Because the acquisition of problem-solving ability requires that students rely on new and important ways of seeing things rather than memorizing the book and notes, some students find the transition more difficult than others. Some students are more able to deal in the abstract, concept-oriented framework than others. Students who have typically relied on "pure memory" for their success will find a need to focus on concepts and problem solving. They may struggle at first, just as they may have struggled with the first word problem in algebra. But the reward for such struggle is 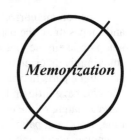 intellectual growth. That's what college is supposed to stimulate. With such growth will come an increased ability to solve a variety of problems beyond genetics. Problem solving is a process, a style, that can be applied to many disciplines. Few people are actually born with the touch of synthetic brilliance. Success comes from probing deeply into a few areas to see how problems are approached in a given discipline. Then, because problems are usually approached in a fairly consistent manner, a given problem-solving approach can often be applied to a variety of activities.

Read ahead. You have been told that it is important to read the assigned material before attending lectures. This allows you to make full use of the information provided in the lecture and to concentrate on those areas that are unclear in the readings. An opportunity is often provided for asking questions. Your questions will be received much more favorably if you can say that after reading the book and listening to the lecture, a particular point is still unclear. It is very likely that your question will be quickly dealt with to your benefit and the benefit of others in the class.

Ask Questions and Don't Tune Out!

How to Study

Genetics is a science that involves symbols (A, b, p), structures (chromosomes, ribosomes, plasmids), and processes (meiosis, replication, translation) that interact in a variety of ways. Models describe the manner in which hereditary units are made, how they function, and how they are transmitted from parent to offspring. Because many parts of the models interact in both time and space, genetics can not be viewed as a discipline filled with facts that should be memorized. Rather, one must be, or become, comfortable with seeking to understand not only the components of the models but also how the models work.

One can memorize the names and shapes of all the parts of an automobile engine, but without studying the interrelationships among the parts in time and space, one will have little understanding of the real nature of the engine. It takes time, work, and patience to see how an engine works, and it will take time, work, and patience to understand genetics.

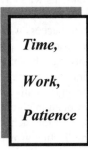

Time, Work, Patience

Don't cram. A successful tennis player doesn't learn to play tennis overnight; therefore, you can't expect to learn genetics under the pressure of night-long cramming. It will be necessary for you to develop and follow a realistic study schedule for genetics as well as the other courses you are taking. It is important that you focus your study periods into intensive but short sessions each day throughout the entire semester (quarter, trimester). Because genetics tests often require you to think "on the spot," it is very important that you get a good night's sleep before each test. Avoid caffeine in the evening before the test because a clear, rested, well-prepared mind will be required.

Study when there are no tests.

Study goals. The instruction of genetics is often divided into large conceptual units. A test usually follows each unit. It will be necessary for you to study genetics on a routine basis long before each test. To do so, set specific study goals. Adhere to these goals and don't let examinations in one course interfere with the study goals of another course. Notice that each course being taken is handled in the same way—study ahead of time and don't cram.

Study each subject at least every other day—especially when there are no tests!

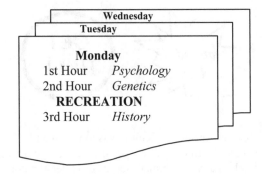

	Wednesday	
	Tuesday	
Monday		
1st Hour	*Psychology*	
2nd Hour	*Genetics*	
RECREATION		
3rd Hour	*History*	

Develop a Realistic Monthly Schedule

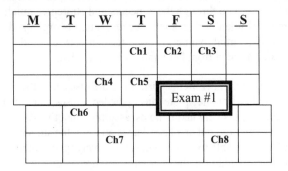

M	T	W	T	F	S	S
			Ch1	Ch2	Ch3	
		Ch4	Ch5			
				Exam #1		
	Ch6					
		Ch7			Ch8	

Develop a Plan for the Semester

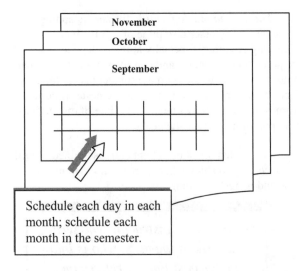

November

October

September

Schedule each day in each month; schedule each month in the semester.

Work the assigned problems. The basic concepts of genetics are really quite straightforward, but there are many examples that apply to these concepts. To help students adjust to the variety of examples and approaches to concepts, instructors often assign practice problems from the back of each chapter. If your instructor has assigned certain problems, finish working them *at least* one week before each examination. Before starting a set of problems, read the chapter carefully and consider the information presented in class.

Suggestions for working problems:

(1) Work the problem without looking at the answer. Commit each answer to paper!

(2) Check your answer in this book.

(3) If incorrect, work the problem again.

(4) If still incorrect, you don't understand the concept.

(5) Reread your lecture notes and the text.

(6) Work the problem again.

(7) If you still don't understand the solution, mark it, and go to the next problem.

In your next study session, return to those problems that you have marked. Expect to make mistakes and learn from those mistakes. Sometimes what is difficult to see one day may be obvious the next. If you are still having problems with a concept, schedule a meeting with your instructor. The problem can, be cleared up in a few minutes.

You will notice that in this book, I have presented the solution to each problem. I provide different ways of looking at some of the problems. Instructors often take a problem directly from those at the end of the chapters or they will modify an existing problem. Reversing the "direction" of a question is a common approach. Instead of giving characteristics of the parents and asking for characteristics of the offspring, the question may provide characteristics of the offspring and ask for

particulars on the parents. Think as you work the problems.

Separate examples from concepts. As mentioned earlier, genetics boils down to a few (perhaps 15 to 20) basic concepts. However, there are many examples that apply to those concepts. Too often, students have trouble separating examples from the concepts. Examples allow you to picture, in concrete terms, various phenomena, but they don't exemplify each phenomenon or concept in its entirety.

Be careful when using old examinations. It is often customary for students to request or otherwise obtain old examinations from previous students. Such a practice is loaded with pitfalls. First, students often, albeit unconsciously, find themselves "second guessing" questions on an upcoming examination. They

> *Old examinations may help, but...*

forget that an examination usually covers only a subset of the available information in a section. Therefore, entire conceptual areas may be available that have not appeared on recent exams.

The reproductions of old examinations are often of poor quality (having been copied and passed around repeatedly), and it is difficult to determine whether the answer provided is correct. In addition, if a question has the same general structure as one on a previous examination but is modified, students often provide an answer for the "old" question rather than the one being asked. Granted, it is of value to see the format of each question and the general emphasis of previous examinations, but remember that each examination is potentially a new production capable of covering areas that have not been tested before. This is especially likely in a course such as genetics for which the material changes very rapidly.

> *Don't try to figure out what will be asked. Study all the material as well as possible.*

Structure of This Book

The intent of this book is to help you understand the concepts of genetics as given in the text and most likely given in the lectures, then to apply these concepts to the solution of all problems and questions at the end of each chapter. Rather than merely providing you with the solutions to the problems, I have tried to walk you through each component of each question so that you can see from where information is obtained and how it can be applied in the solution. At the beginning of each chapter

Students: Read All of This Section First!!!

is a section that relates general concept areas to particular problems. This should help you practice certain conceptual areas as needed.

> **Master each listed term, its context, and related examples.**

Listing of terms and concepts. Understanding the vocabulary of a discipline is essential to understanding the discipline. Throughout the text by Klug et al., you will find terms in bold print. Those words, plus others have been listed at the front of each chapter in this book. In some cases, certain terms are identified (*) that deserve special attention. Be certain to master the meaning of each listed term as to its precise meaning, the context in which it is presented, and examples relating to each.

Use the listings as checklists to make certain that you understand the meaning of each term in each chapter. Notice that the various terms are not redefined. It is important that you use the text for the original definitions.

> **Understand the words and phrases of the discipline.**

Solved problems and discussion questions. Each of the problems at the end of each chapter is solved from a beginner's point of view. There are other features of this section. Many of the answers to the questions and problems will refer you to the text. Be certain that you fully understand the solution to each of the questions suggested or assigned by your instructor.

Chapter 1: Introduction to Genetics

Concept Areas	Corresponding Problems
Mendelism	1, 3, 4
Homologous Chromosomes	6
Chromosome Theory of Inheritance	1, 2, 6
Central Dogma of Molecular Genetics	5, 7, 8, 9
Model Organisms and Methods	10, 14
Genetics and Social Issues	11, 12, 13, 15, 16

Structures and Processes Checklist – Significant concepts that deserve special attention are identified with a "∗".

(check topic when mastered – provide examples where appropriate – understand the context of each entry)

- ○ **Historical**
  - ○ HSD*
  - ○ deCODE*
  - ○ privacy
  - ○ Hippocratic School
  - ○ Aristotle
  - ○ Modern Biology
  - ○ epigenesis*
  - ○ preformation
  - ○ homunculus
  - ○ cell theory
  - ○ spontaneous generation
  - ○ Charles Darwin
  - ○ natural selection*
  - ○ chromosome theory*
  - ○ genetics*

- ○ **Mendel to DNA**
  - ○ transmission of traits
  - ○ genetics*
  - ○ chromosome theory*
  - ○ Mendel and meiosis
  - ○ diploid number (2*n*)*
  - ○ mitosis and meiosis*
  - ○ haploid number (*n*)*
  - ○ genetic variation*
  - ○ mutation
  - ○ allele*
  - ○ phenotype*
  - ○ genotype*
- ○ **Era of Molecular Genetics**
  - ○ DNA, RNA
  - ○ nucleotides

- gene expression
- DNA to phenotype*
- transcription*
- messenger RNA (mRNA)
- ribosome
- translation*
- genetic code*
- codon
- proteins
- enzymes
- genotype to phenotype*
- sickle-cell anemia*
- hemoglobin
- glutamic acid to valine
- **Recombinant DNA Technology***
  - DNA cloning
  - restriction enzymes*
  - clone
  - vectors
  - genome

- **Impact of Biotechnology**
  - transgenic
  - herbicide-resistant crops
  - genetics and medicine
- **Genomics, Proteomics...***
  - genomics
  - proteomics
  - bioinformatics
- **Model Organisms***
  - *Drosophila melanogester*
  - *Mus musculus*
  - *Saccharomyces cerevisiae*
  - T phages
  - lambda phage
  - *Caenorhabditis elegans*
  - *Arabidopsis thaliana*
  - *Danio rerio*
  - *E. coli*
- **Age of Genetics**
  - Nobel prizes
  - genetics and society*

F1-1 Simple diagram of the relationships among major components of the *trinity of molecular genetics*

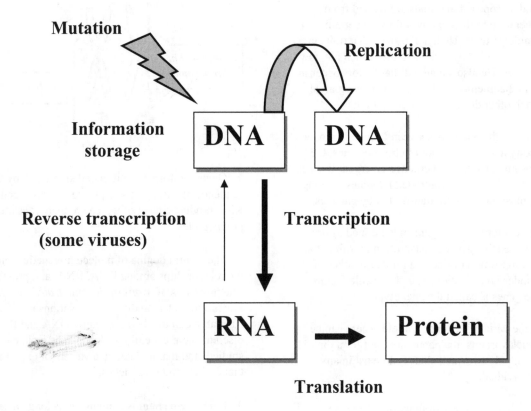

Chapter 1 Introduction to Genetics

Solutions to Problems and Discussion Questions

1. Mendel proposed that traits are passed from one generation to the next by following certain predictable patterns. He hypothesized that traits in peas are controlled by discrete units, which are now called genes. He also suggested that factors occur in pairs and that members of each gene pair separate from each other during gamete formation.

2. Based on the parallels between Mendel's model of heredity and the behavior of chromosomes, the chromosome theory of inheritance emerged. It states that inherited traits are controlled by genes residing on chromosomes that are transmitted by gametes.

3. The genotype of an organism is defined as its specific allelic or genetic constitution or, often, the allelic composition of one or a limited number of genes under investigation. The observable feature of those genes is called the phenotype.

4. A gene variant is called an allele. There can be many such variants in a population, but for a diploid organism, only two such alleles can exist in any given individual.

5. Genes have a variety of functions. Because proteins can contain up to 20 different amino acids, each being structurally unique, a vast amount of functional variation is possible. In addition, proteins can engage in a variety of enzymatic activities. DNA is made up of only six components (sugar, phosphate, and four bases) arranged in a rather monotonous, linear fashion. It seemed likely that proteins, given their cellular abundance and versatility, should be the genetic material.

6. *Genes*, linear sequences of nucleotides, usually exert their influence by producing polypeptides through the process of transcription and translation. Genes are the functional units of heredity. They associate, sometimes with proteins, to form *chromosomes*. During the cell cycle, chromosomes, and therefore genes, are duplicated by a variety of enzymes so that daughter cells inherit copies of the parental hereditary information. Genes of eukaryotes and prokaryotes are composed of DNA.

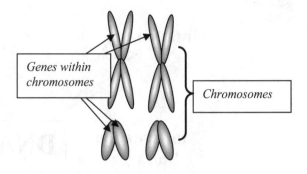

Genes within chromosomes

Chromosomes

7. Genetic information is encoded in DNA by the sequence of bases. This sequence is transcribed into RNA products, most of which are then translated into polypeptides.

8. The central dogma of molecular genetics refers to the relationships among DNA, RNA, and proteins. The processes of *transcription* and *translation* are integral to understanding these relationships. See F1-1 above in this book. Because DNA and RNA are discrete chemical entities, they can be isolated, studied, and manipulated in a variety of experiments that define modern genetics.

9. If a protein chain is 5 amino acids long, at each position there can be 20 amino acids; therefore, there would be 20^5 different possible combinations.

10. Restriction enzymes (endonucleases) cut double-stranded DNA at particular base sequences. Often, short single-stranded overhangs are generated so that ends from one fragment can anneal with ends from another (assuming the same enzyme is used). When a vector is cleaved with the same enzyme, complementary ends are created such that ends, regardless of their origin, can be combined and ligated to form intact double-stranded structures. Such recombinant forms are often useful for industrial, research, and/or pharmaceutical efforts.

11. In the past 50 years, traditional transmission, cytological, and molecular genetics have provided an understanding of many aspects of both plant and animal biology, including development of

4

pest-resistant crops and identification of hazardous organisms in our food (*E. coli,* for example). Recently, biotechnology has allowed genes to be moved in a variety of ways to generate transgenic plants. Such organisms can be engineered to increase their ecological breadth, disease resistance, and/or nutrient value. Wheat, rice, corn, beans, and cassava are being modified to enhance nutritional value by increasing vitamin and mineral content.

12. Unique transgenic plants and animals can be patented, as ruled by the United States Supreme Court in 1980. Supporters of organismic patenting argue that it is needed to encourage innovation and allow the costs of discovery to be recovered. Capital investors assume that there is a likely chance that their investments will yield positive returns. Others argue that natural substances should not be privately owned and that once they are owned by a small number of companies, free enterprise will be stifled.

13. Some mechanism should be in place to protect the investments of individuals and institutions that develop needed and useful products. However, safeguards, both ethical and economic, need to be developed to ensure that relatively free and fair access exists when vital issues are in question. Any mechanism needs to protect investors as well as consumers.

14. Model organisms are not only useful, but also necessary for understanding genes that influence human diseases. Given that many genetic/molecular systems are highly conserved across broad phylogenetic lines, what is learned in one organism is usually applied to all organisms. In addition, most model organisms have peculiarities, such as ease of growth, "understandable genetics"; or abundant offspring, that make their use straightforward and especially informative in genetic studies.

15. This question is open to many "answers" depending on the individual. Although it may be difficult to put yourself in this position, consider not only what your decision would be, but also why you would make such a decision. Often, as a person ages, his or her perspective changes; for instance, how would the possibility of children under your care influence your decision?

16. For approximately 60 years, discoveries in genetics have guided our understanding of living systems, aided rational drug design, and dominated many social discussions. Genetics provides the framework for universal biological processes and helps explain species stability and diversity. Given the central focus of genetics in so many of life's processes, it is understandable why so many genetic scientists have been awarded the Nobel Prize.

Chapter 2: Mitosis and Meiosis

Concept Areas	Corresponding Problems
Cell Structure	2
Homology of Chromosomes	1, 3, 4, 6, 12, 23
Cell Division	1, 7, 8
Mitosis	5, 8, 9, 15, 16, 24, 30
Meiosis	9, 10, 11, 12, 13, 14, 15, 16, 17, 18, 19, 20, 25, 26, 27, 28, 29, 30
Chromosome Structure	19, 21, 22

Structures and Processes Checklist – Significant concepts that deserve special attention are identified with a "*".

(check topic when mastered – provide examples where appropriate – understand the context of each entry)

- **Mitosis, Meiosis**
  - sexual reproduction
  - gametes
  - spores
- **Cell Structure**
  - plasma membrane
  - cell wall
  - glycocalyx
  - cell coat
  - receptor molecules
  - eukaryotic cells*
  - nucleus
  - chromatin
  - chromosomes
  - nucleolus
  - rRNA

- nucleolus organizer region
- NOR
- prokaryotic cells*
- nucleoid
- cytoplasm
- endoplasmic reticulum
- ER
- mRNA
- mitochondria
- chloroplasts
- endosymbiotic hypothesis*
- centrioles
- spindle fibers
- **Homologous Pairs (Diploid)***
  - metacentric
  - submetacentric

Chapter 2 Mitosis and Meiosis

- o acrocentric
- o telocentric
- o centromere
- o p arm
- o q arm
- o diploid number (2*n*)*
- o homologous chromosomes*
- o karyotype
- o sister chromatids*
- o haploid number (*n*)*
- o locus (loci)
- o biparental inheritance
- o alleles*
- o sex-determining chromosomes
- o **Mitosis Partitions Chromosomes***
  - o zygotes
  - o karyokinesis
  - o cytokinesis
  - o interphase*
  - o S phase*
  - o G1 (gap I)*
  - o G2 (gap II)*
  - o DNA replication*
  - o M phase*
  - o G0 stage
  - o prophase
  - o centrosome
  - o sister chromatids*
  - o cohesion
- o prometaphase
- o metaphase*
- o kinetochore
- o shugoshin
- o anaphase*
- o daughter chromosome
- o molecular motors
- o telophase*
- o cytokinesis
- o cell plate
- o middle lamella
- o cell furrow
- o cell-cycle regulation*
- o checkpoints*
- o *cell division cycle* mutations*
- o *cdc*
- o kinases
- o potential malignancy*
- o **Meiosis Creates Haploid Gametes***
  - o meiosis*
  - o crossing over*
  - o prophase I*
  - o sister chromatids*
  - o synapsis*
  - o bivalent*
  - o tetrad*
  - o chiasma*
  - o nonsister chromatids*
  - o metaphase I*

- o side-by-side alignment*
- o anaphase I*
- o disjunction*
- o nondisjunction*
- o telophase I*
- o second meiotic division*
- o meiosis II*
- o prophase II*
- o anaphase II*
- o telophase II*
- o haploid state*
- o **Development of Gametes***
  - o spermatogenesis*
  - o spermatogonium*
  - o primary spermatocyte*
  - o secondary spermatocyte*
  - o spermatid*
- o spermiogenesis
- o spermatozoa
- o sperm
- o oogenesis*
- o ova (ovum)
- o first polar body*
- o secondary oocyte*
- o second polar body*
- o ootid*
- o **Meiosis and Sexual Reproduction***
  - o diploid organisms*
  - o genetic variation*
  - o sporophyte
  - o gametophyte
- o **Electron Microscopy**
  - o dispersed chromatin
  - o folded-fiber model
  - o 5000-fold compaction

F2-1 Diagram illustrating relationships among stages of interphase. Also illustrated are chromosomes, chromosome number, and structure in an organism with a diploid chromosome number of 4 (2*n* = 4). Individual chromosomes cannot be seen at interphase; therefore, the chromosomes pictured here are hypothetical. In mitosis, the chromosome number does not change even though the DNA content doubles during the S phase. The chromosomes become doubled structures as a result of the S phase.

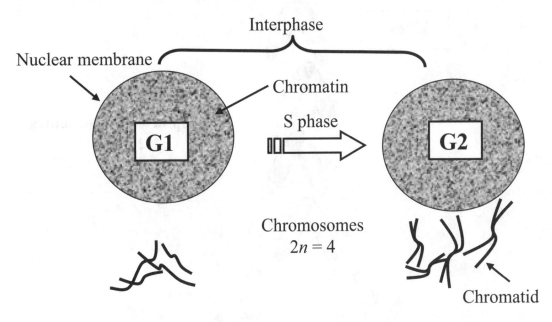

F2-2 Important nomenclature referring to chromosomes and genes in an organism where the diploid chromosome number is 4 (2*n* = 4). There are two pairs of chromosomes: one large metacentric and one small telocentric. Sister chromatids are identical to each other, whereas homologous chromosomes are similar to each other in terms of overall size, centromere location, function, and other factors described in the text.

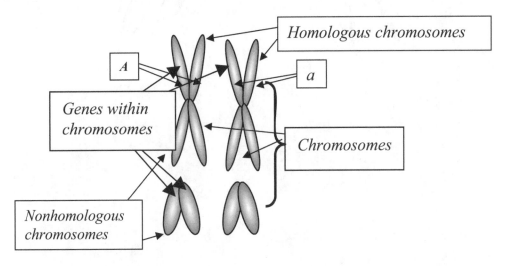

F2-3 Illustration of chromosomes of mitotic cells in an organism with a chromosome number of 4 ($2n = 4$).

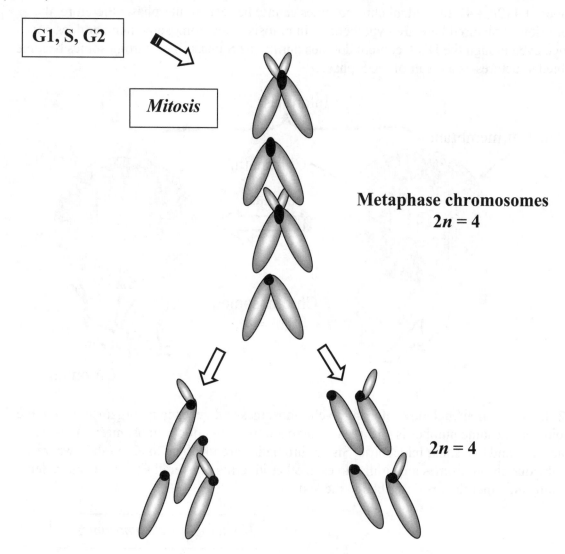

G1, S, G2

Mitosis

Metaphase chromosomes
$2n = 4$

$2n = 4$

F2-4 Illustration of chromosomes of meiotic cells in an organism with a chromosome number of 4 ($2n = 4$).

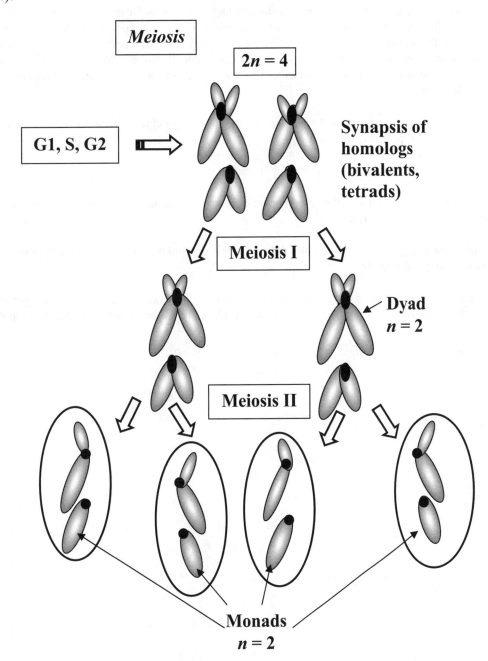

Answers to Now Solve This

2-1. The first sentence tells you that $2n = 16$ and it is a question about mitosis. Because each chromosome in prophase is doubled (having gone through an S phase) and is visible at the end of prophase, there should be 32 chromatids. Because the centromeres divide and what were previously sister chromatids migrate to opposite poles during anaphase, there should be 16 chromosomes moving to each pole. If you refer to F2-2, you will see an example with $2n = 4$ and that there are four doubled chromosomes in prophase. Notice that there are eight chromatids visible at late prophase.

2-2. Look carefully at F2-4 in this book and notice that for a cell with four chromosomes, there are two tetrads each composed of a homologous pair of chromosomes.

(a) If there are 16 chromosomes, there should be eight tetrads.

(b) Also note that after meiosis I and in the second meiotic prophase, there are as many dyads as there are pairs of chromosomes. There will be eight dyads.

(c) Because the monads migrate to opposite poles during meiosis II (from the separation of dyads), there should be eight monads migrating to *each* pole.

2-3. Not necessarily. If crossing over occurred in meiosis I, then the chromatids in the secondary oocyte are not identical. Once they separate during meiosis II, dissimilar chromatids reside in the ootid and the second polar body.

Chapter 2   Mitosis and Meiosis

Solutions to Problems and Discussion Questions

1. **(a)** When somatic cells from the same species are examined, they contain the same number of chromosomes and the lengths and centromere placements of nearly all such chromosomes can be matched into pairs. **(b)** The initiation and completion of DNA synthesis can be detected by the incorporation of labeled precursors into DNA. DNA content in a G2 nucleus is twice that of a G1 nucleus. **(c)** If the fibers comprising the mitotic chromosomes are loosened, they reveal fibers like those of interphase chromatin. Electron microscopic observations indicate that mitotic chromosomes are in varying states of extensively folded structures derived from chromatin.

2. **(a)** During interphase of the cell cycle (mitotic and meiotic), chromosomes are not condensed and are in a genetically active, spread out form. In this condition, chromosomes are not visible as individual structures under the microscope (light or electron). See F2-1 for a sketch of what *chromatin* might look like. Chromatin contains the genetic material that is responsible for maintaining hereditary information (from one cell to daughter cells and from one generation to the next) and production of the phenotype.

(b) The *nucleolus* (pl. *nucleoli*) is a structure that is produced by activity of the nucleolar organizer region in eukaryotes. Composed of ribosomal RNA and protein, it is the structure for the production of ribosomes. Some nuclei have more than one nucleolus. Nucleoli are not present during mitosis or meiosis because in the condensed state of chromosomes, there is little or no RNA synthesis.

(c) The *ribosome* is the structure where various RNAs, enzymes, and other molecular species assemble the primary sequence of a protein. That is, amino acids are placed in order as specified by messenger RNA. Ribosomes are relatively nonspecific in that virtually any ribosome can be used in the translation of any mRNA. The structure and function of the ribosome will be described in greater detail in later chapters of the text.

(d) The *mitochondrion* (pl. *mitochondria*) is a membrane-bound structure located in the cytoplasm of eukaryotic cells. It is the site of oxidative phosphorylation and production of relatively large amounts of ATP. It is the trapping of energy in ATP that drives many important metabolic processes in living systems.

(e) The *centriole* is a cytoplasmic structure involved (through the formation of spindle fibers) in the migration of chromosomes during mitosis and meiosis of animal cells.

(f) The *centromere* serves as an attachment point for sister chromatids (see F2-3, F2-4) and a region where spindle fibers attach to chromosomes (kinetochore). The centromere divides during mitosis and meiosis II, thus aiding in the partitioning of chromosomal material to daughter cells. Failure of centromeres or spindle fibers to function properly may result in nondisjunction.

3. One of the most important concepts to be gained from this chapter is the relationship that exists among chromosomes in a single cell. Chromosomes that are homologous normally share many properties, including the following:

Overall length. Look carefully at the figures above to see that each cell, prior to anaphase I, contains two chromosomes in which a homolog is of approximately the same overall length.

Position of the centromere (metacentric, submetacentric, acrocentric, telocentric). Again, look carefully at F2-2 and F2-3. Notice that in each if there is one metacentric chromosome, there will be another metacentric chromosome.

Banding patterns. Using various cytological techniques, bands can be induced in chromosomes. Homologous chromosomes of pair #1, for example, will have the same banding pattern. Although the overall length of chromosome pairs #16 and #17 appears to be the same, the banding patterns of these nonhomologous chromosomes will be different.

Sister chromatids have identical banding patterns, as would be expected because sister chromatids are, with the exception of mutation, identical copies of each other. We would expect that homologous chromosomes would have banding patterns that are very similar (but not identical) because homologous chromosomes are genetically similar but not genetically identical.

Type and location of genes. Notice in F2-2 that a locus signifies the location of a gene along a chromosome. What that really means is that for each characteristic specified by a gene, such as blood type, eye color, or skin pigmentation, there are genes located along chromosomes. The *order* of such loci is identical in homologous chromosomes, but the genes themselves, while being in the same order, may not be identical. Look carefully at the inset (box) in the upper portion of F2-2 and see that there are alternative forms of genes,

A and *a*, at the same location along the chromosome. *A* and *a* are located at the same place and specify the same *characteristic* (eye color, for example), but there are slightly different manifestations of eye color (*brown* vs. *blue,* for example). Just as an individual may inherit gene *A* from the father and gene *a* from the mother, each zygote inherits one homolog of each pair from the father and one homolog of each pair from the mother.

Autoradiographic pattern. Homologous chromosomes tend to replicate during the same time of S phase.

Diploidy is a term often used in conjunction with the symbol 2*n*. It means that both members of a homologous pair of chromosomes are present. Refer to F2-1 in this book. Notice that during mitosis, the normal chromosome complement is 2*n* or diploid. In humans, the diploid chromosome number is 46, while in *Drosophila melanogaster* it is 8. The text lists the *haploid* chromosome number for a variety of species.

The haploid chromosome number is one-half the diploid number. However, it is very important to realize that *haploidy* specifically refers to the fact that each haploid cell contains *one chromosome of each homologous pair of chromosomes.*

Compare the nuclear contents of a spermatid and a cell at zygonema in the text. Note that each spermatid contains one member of each of the original chromosome pairs (seen at zygonema). Haploidy is usually symbolized as *n*.

The change from a diploid (2*n*) to haploid (*n*) occurs during *reduction division* when tetrads become dyads during meiosis I. Referring to the number of human chromosomes, the primary spermatocyte (2*n* = 46) becomes two secondary spermatocytes each with *n* = 23.

4. As you examine the criteria for *homology* in question 2 above, you can see that overall length and centromere position are but two factors required for homology. Most importantly, genetic content in nonhomologous chromosomes is expected to be quite different. Other factors including banding pattern and time of replication during S phase would also be expected to vary among nonhomologous chromosomes.

5. Because a major section of Chapter 2 deals with mitosis, it would be best to deal with this question by reading the appropriate section in the text and examining the corresponding figures. Understanding mitosis and all the related terms is essential for an understanding of genetics.

6. Refer to the text figures for an explanation. Notice the different anaphase shapes of chromosomes as they

move to the poles: metacentric (a), submetacentric (b), acrocentric (c), and telocentric (d).

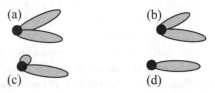

7. Because of a cell wall around the plasma membrane in plants, a cell plate, which was laid down during anaphase, becomes the middle lamella where primary and secondary layers of the cell wall are deposited. No such structure is seen in animal cells.

8. Carefully read the section on mitosis and cell division in the text. Major divisions of the cell cycle include interphase and mitosis. Interphase is composed of three phases: G1, S, and G2. (Some cells have a temporary or permanent G0 phase between G1 and S.) During the S phase, chromosomal DNA doubles. Karyokinesis involves nuclear division, whereas cytokinesis involves division of the cytoplasm. Refer to F2-1 for information pertaining to the interphase. Refer to the text figures for a diagram of mitosis. Notice that in contrast to meiosis, there is no pairing of homologous chromosomes in mitosis and the chromosome number does not change.

9. Compared with mitosis, which maintains a chromosomal constancy, meiosis provides for a reduction in chromosome number and an opportunity for exchange of genetic material between homologous chromosomes. In mitosis, there is no change in chromosome number or kind in the two daughter cells, whereas in meiosis, numerous potentially different haploid (*n*) cells are produced. During oogenesis, only one of the four meiotic products is functional; however, four of the four meiotic products of spermatogenesis are potentially functional.

10. (a) *Synapsis* is the point-by-point pairing of homologous chromosomes during prophase of meiosis I.

(b) *Bivalents* are those structures formed by the synapsis of homologous chromosomes. In other words, there are two chromosomes (and four chromatids) that make up a bivalent. If an organism has a diploid chromosome number of 46, then there will be 23 bivalents in meiosis I.

(c) *Chiasmata* is the plural form of chiasma and refers to the structure, when viewed microscopically, of crossed chromatids. Notice the figures in the text showing the exchange of chromatid pieces in diplonema and diakinesis.

(d) *Crossing over* is the exchange of genetic material between chromatids. If there are allelic differences between the two homologs, crossing over results in genetic recombination. It is a method of providing genetic variation through the breaking and rejoining of chromatids.

(e) Examine F2-1 in this book. Notice that *sister chromatids* are "post-S phase" structures of replicated chromosomes. Sister chromatids are genetically identical (except where mutations have occurred) and are originally attached to the same centromere. Identify sister chromatids in the figures in the text. Note that sister chromatids separate from each other during anaphase of mitosis and anaphase II of meiosis.

(f) *Tetrads* are synapsed homologous chromosomes thereby composed of four chromatids. There are as many tetrads as the haploid chromosome number.

(g) Actually, each tetrad is made of two dyads that separate from each other during anaphase I of meiosis. Note that *dyads* are composed of two chromatids joined by a centromere.

(h) At anaphase II of meiosis, the centromeres divide and sister chromatids (*monads*) go to opposite poles.

11. Sister chromatids are genetically identical, except where mutations may have occurred during DNA replication. Nonsister chromatids are genetically similar if on homologous chromosomes and genetically dissimilar if on nonhomologous chromosomes. If crossing over occurs, then chromatids attached to the same centromere may no longer be identical.

12. During meiosis I, the chromosome number is reduced to haploid complements. This is achieved by synapsis of homologous chromosomes and their subsequent separation. It would seem to be more mechanically difficult for genetically identical daughters to form from mitosis if homologous chromosomes paired. By having chromosomes unpaired at metaphase of mitosis, only centromere division is required for daughter cells to eventually receive identical chromosomal complements.

13. Examine appropriate figures in the text. Notice that major differences include the sex in which each occurs, and that the distribution of cytoplasm is unequal in oogenesis but considered to be equal in the products of spermatogenesis. Chromosomal behavior is the same in spermatogenesis and oogenesis except that the nuclear

activity in oogenesis is "off-center," thereby producing first and second polar bodies by unequal cytoplasmic division.

In humans, each spermatogonium and primary spermatocyte produces four spermatids, whereas each oogonium and primary oocyte produces one ootid. Because early development occurs in the absence of outside nutrients, it is likely that the unequal distribution of cytoplasm in oogenesis evolved to provide sufficient information and nutrients to support development until the transcriptional activities of the zygotic nucleus begin to provide products.

Polar bodies probably represent nonfunctional by-products of such evolution.

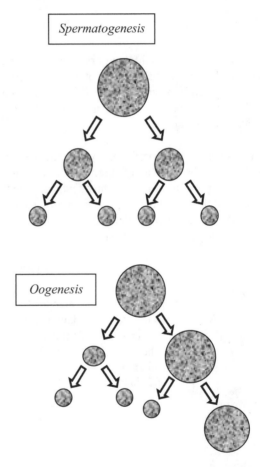

14. This answer contains several parts. First, through independent assortment of chromosomes at anaphase I of meiosis, daughter cells (secondary spermatocytes and secondary oocytes) may contain different sets of maternally and paternally derived chromosomes. Examine the diagram that follows. Notice that there are several ways in which the maternally and paternally derived chromosomes may align. Can you calculate the probability of all the maternally derived chromosomes going to the "right-hand" pole? Second, crossing over, which happens at a much higher frequency in meiotic cells as compared to mitotic cells, allows maternally and paternally derived chromosomes to exchange segments, thereby increasing the likelihood that daughter cells (that is, secondary spermatocytes and secondary oocytes) are genetically unique.

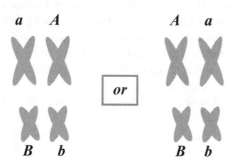

a   A   A   a

B   b   B   b

or

Notice that there are two different orientations of tetrads in meiosis. Independent assortment of nonhomologous chromosomes adds to genetic variability. Daughter cells resulting from the process of mitosis are usually genetically identical.

15. This question specifically tests your understanding of meiosis and the behavior of chromosomes during anaphase. For this question, you must first visualize the alignment of the three homologous chromosome pairs C1/C2, M1/M2, and S1/S2 in mitosis where there is no synapsis of homologous chromosomes.

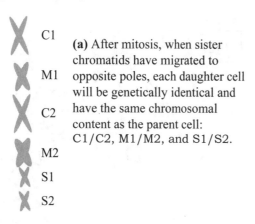

C1
M1
C2
M2
S1
S2

(a) After mitosis, when sister chromatids have migrated to opposite poles, each daughter cell will be genetically identical and have the same chromosomal content as the parent cell: C1/C2, M1/M2, and S1/S2.

(b) The first meiotic metaphase will have the following configuration:

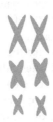

Label each chromosome according to the symbols in part **(a)** above.

(c) For the haploid products of the cell in part **(b)**, there are eight possibilities, depending on the alignment of the homologous chromosomes:

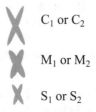

C_1 or C_2

M_1 or M_2

S_1 or S_2

16. If there are eight combinations possible in part **(c)** in the previous problem, there would be 16 combinations with the addition of another chromosome pair.

17. 50, 50, 50, 100, 200

18. One-half of each tetrad will have a maternal homolog: $(1/2)^{10}$.

19. In prophase I, homologous duplicated chromosomes pair in a process called synapsis. Each synapsed pair of homologs is initially called a bivalent. As condensation occurs, tetrads are formed consisting of two pairs of sister chromatids. As prophase I progresses, sister chromatids pull apart, but with one or more sections of the chromatids intertwined forming a chiasma. It is likely that genetic exchange (crossing over) occurs at such points. At the end of prophase I, the nucleolus and nuclear envelope break down, and the centromeres of each tetrad attach to spindle fibers.

20. In angiosperms, meiosis results in the formation of microspores (male) and megaspores (female), which give rise to the haploid male and female gametophyte stage. Micro- and megagametophytes produce the pollen and the ovules, respectively. Following fertilization, the sporophyte is formed.

21. The transition from chromatin to individual chromosomes occurs at the beginning of mitosis (or meiosis). During this time, chromatin fibers fold up and condense into the typical mitotic chromosome. The *folded-fiber model* depicts this transition.

22. The folded-fiber model is based on each chromatid consisting of a single fiber wound like a skein of yarn. Each fiber consists of DNA and protein. A coiling process occurs during the transition of interphase chromatin to more condensed chromosomes during prophase of mitosis or meiosis. Such condensation leads to a 5000-fold contraction in the length of the DNA within each chromatid. The transition is at the end of interphase and the beginning of prophase when the chromosomes are in the condensation process. This eventually leads to the typically shortened and "fattened" metaphase chromosome.

23. They would probably be homologous chromosomes and contain similar (but not identical) genetic information. Their centromeres would most likely be in the same position relative to chromosome arm lengths, and any physical characteristics such as secondary constrictions or bands would be similar. They would have a similar sequence of nitrogenous bases. They would most likely replicate synchronously during the S phase of the cell cycle.

24. Duplicated chromosomes A^m, A^p, B^m, B^p, C^m, and C^p will align at metaphase, with the centromeres dividing and sister chromatids going to opposite poles at anaphase.

25. Side-by-side alignment of A^m, A^p, B^m, B^p, C^m, and C^p will occur in various arrangements at metaphase I. Eight possible combinations of products will occur at the completion of anaphase: A^m, B^p, C^m, for example (each with sister chromatids). In other words, after meiosis I, the two product cells would be as follows: A^m or A^p, B^m or B^p, C^m or C^p.

26. As long as you have accounted for eight possible combinations in the previous problem, there would be no new ones added in this problem.

27. Eight (2 X 2 X 2) combinations are possible.

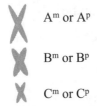

A^m or A^p

B^m or B^p

C^m or C^p

28. See the products of nondisjunction of chromosome C at the end of meiosis I as follows:

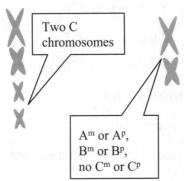

Two C chromosomes

A^m or A^p, B^m or B^p, no C^m or C^p

At the end of meiosis II, assuming that, as the problem states, the C chromosomes separate as dyads instead of monads during meiosis II, you would have monads for the A and B chromosomes and dyads (from the cell on the left) for both C chromosomes as one possibility.

However, another possibility exists, as shown next for the products of meiosis II:

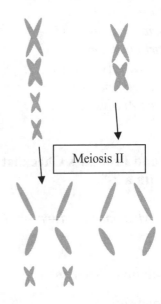

Meiosis II

29. Taking this question exactly as it is described— nondisjunction of the C chromosome at meiosis I and again, nondisjunction of the same chromosome at meiosis II, you will end up, after fertilization, with the following combinations:

zygote 1:   two copies of chromosome A
               two copies of chromosome B
               five copies of chromosome C

zygotes 2–4:   two copies of chromosome A
               two copies of chromosome B
               one copy of chromosome C

Under the second possibility described in problem 28, one would expect the following zygotes after fertilization:

zygotes 1–2:   two copies of chromosome A
               two copies of chromosome B
               three copies of chromosome C

zygotes 3–4:   two copies of chromosome A
               two copies of chromosome B
               one copy of chromosome C

30. 0.72 picograms; 0.36 picograms; 0.72 picograms

Chapter 3: Mendelian Genetics

Concept Areas	Corresponding Problems
Mendel's Postulates	1, 4, 5, 8, 9, 11, 22
Monohybrid Crosses	2, 3, 4, 7, 11
Homology	10
Dihybrid Crosses	6, 7, 8, 12, 14, 15, 26
Trihybrid Crosses	13, 18, 19, 20
Independent Assortment	6, 7, 8, 12, 14, 15, 25
Chi-Square Analysis	1, 16, 17, 27
Pedigree Analysis	1, 21, 22, 23, 24

Structures and Processes Checklist – Significant concepts that deserve special attention are identified with a "*".

(check topic when mastered – provide examples where appropriate – understand the context of each entry)

- **Transmission Genetics**
  - *Pisum sativum*
  - Gregor Johann Mendel
  - 1866
  - units of inheritance*
- **Experimental Approach**
  - patterns of inheritance*
  - artificial hybridization
  - contrasting pairs of traits
- **Monohybrid Cross***
  - one trait
  - selfing
  - parental generation
  - first filial generation
  - second filial generation
  - reciprocal cross

- **Mendel's Postulates***
  - unit factors in pairs
  - dominance/recessiveness
  - segregation
  - terminology*
  - phenotype*
  - genes*
  - alleles*
  - genotype*
  - homozygous*
  - heterozygous*
  - Punnett squares*
  - testcross: one character*
- **Dihybrid Cross***
  - unique F_2 ratio
  - Mendel's fourth postulate

- o independent assortment*
- o product law*
- o Mendel's wrinkled peas
- o 9:3:3:1 dihybrid ratio*
- o testcross: two characters*
- o **Tribybrid Cross***
  - o multiple traits
  - o forked-line method
  - o branch diagram
- o **Rediscovery of Mendel's Work***
  - o continuous variation
  - o Charles Darwin
  - o discontinuous variation
  - o chromosome theory*
  - o Flemming
  - o de Vries, Correns, Tschermak
- o **Correlations***
  - o Mendel's unit factors*
  - o chromosomes during meiosis*
  - o diploid number ($2n$)*
  - o maternal parent
  - o paternal parent
  - o homologous chromosomes*
- o **Independent Assortment***
  - o extensive genetic variation
  - o 2^n*

- o Tay Sachs disease
- o molecular basis
- o **Laws of Probability***
  - o product law*
  - o sum law*
- o **Chi–Square Analysis***
  - o chance deviation
  - o null hypothesis*
  - o degrees of freedom (df)*
  - o probability value (p)*
  - o interpreting probability values*
  - o significant difference*
- o **Pedigrees***
  - o conventions*
  - o consanguineous*
  - o sibs, siblings
  - o sibship line
  - o identical twins*
  - o monozygotic
  - o fraternal twins*
  - o dizygotic
  - o proband (p)
  - o albinism
  - o familial hypercholesterolemia
  - o LDL

F3-1 Illustration of the union of maternal and paternal genes (*A* and *a*) to give two genes in the zygote. Mendelian "unit factors" occur in pairs in diploid organisms. Dominant genes are often given the uppercase letter for their symbol, whereas the lowercase letter is often used to symbolize the recessive gene.

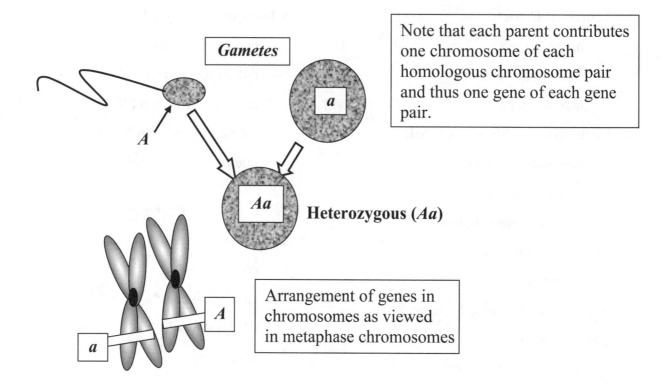

Gametes

Note that each parent contributes one chromosome of each homologous chromosome pair and thus one gene of each gene pair.

Heterozygous (*Aa*)

Arrangement of genes in chromosomes as viewed in metaphase chromosomes

F3-2 Critical symbolism associated with genes and chromosomes. Below are positioned two different gene pairs (*Aa* and *Bb*) on nonhomologous chromosomes. Note that with two different gene pairs, two different characteristics may be involved, such as seed shape (*A* and *a*) and seed color (*B* and *b*).

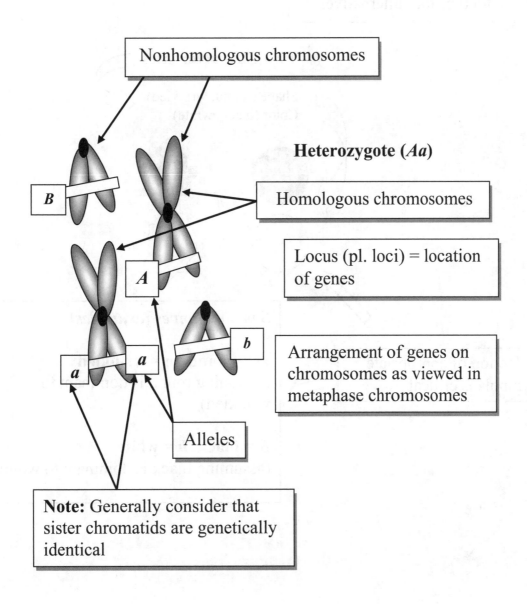

Nonhomologous chromosomes

Heterozygote (*Aa*)

Homologous chromosomes

B

Locus (pl. loci) = location of genes

A

b

Arrangement of genes on chromosomes as viewed in metaphase chromosomes

a *a*

Alleles

Note: Generally consider that sister chromatids are genetically identical

F3-3 One of the most important concepts for this section is illustrated in the figure below. Two gene pairs (*W* and *B*) are presented, each representing a different characteristic: seed shape (*W* or *w*) and seed color (*B* or *b*). Different gene pairs may influence completely different characteristics (as indicated here) or the same characteristic (described in Chapter 4).

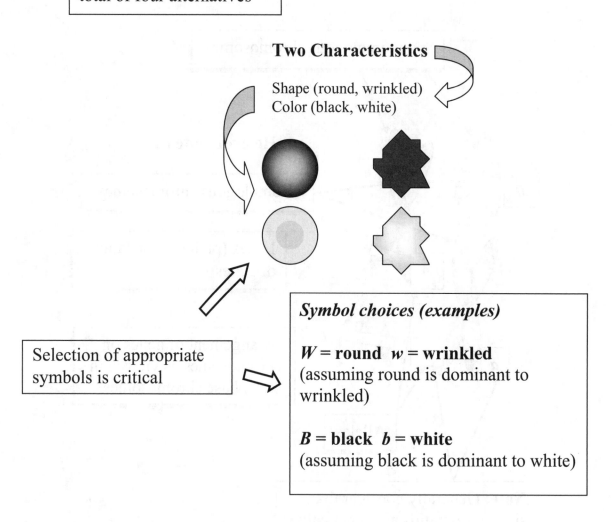

Two characteristics but a total of four alternatives

Two Characteristics

Shape (round, wrinkled)
Color (black, white)

Selection of appropriate symbols is critical

Symbol choices (examples)

W = **round** *w* = **wrinkled**
(assuming round is dominant to wrinkled)

B = **black** *b* = **white**
(assuming black is dominant to white)

Chapter 3 Mendelian Genetics

Answers to Now Solve This

3-1. First, read the entire question and note that you are to determine the pattern of inheritance for "checkered and plain." Notice that there is reference to one characteristic, *pattern*, with two alternatives, checkered vs. plain. We should consider this a monohybrid condition unless complications arise. Assignment of symbols:

P = checkered; p = plain.

Checkered is tentatively assigned the dominant function because in a casual examination of the data, especially cross (b), we see that checkered types are more likely to be produced than plain types.

> Cross (a):
>
> $PP \times PP$ or $PP \times Pp$

> Cross (b):
>
> $PP \times pp$

This assignment seems reasonable because among 38 offspring, no plain types are produced.

Cross (c): Because all the offspring from this cross are plain, there is no doubt that the genotype of both parents is *pp*.

Genotypes of all individuals:

	F_1 Progeny	
P₁ Cross	Checkered	Plain
(a) $PP \times PP$	PP	
$PP \times Pp$	PP, Pp	
(b) $PP \times pp$	Pp	
(c) $pp \times pp$		pp

If you crossed the F_1 generation from cross (b), you would form ¾ checkered and ¼ plain.

3-2. Symbolism as before:

w = wrinkled seeds	g = green cotyledons
W = round seeds	G = yellow cotyledons

Examine each characteristic (seed shape vs. cotyledon color) separately.

(a) Notice a 3:1 ratio for seed shape; therefore, $Ww \times Ww$, and no green cotyledons; therefore, $GG \times GG$ or $GG \times Gg$. Putting the two characteristics together gives

$WwGG \times WwGG$

      or

$WwGG \times WwGg$

(b) Notice a 1:1 ratio for seed shape (8/16 wrinkled and 8/16 round) and a 3:1 ratio for cotyledon color (12/16 yellow and 4/16 green). Therefore, the answer is

$WwGg \times wwGg$

23

(c) This is a typical 1:1:1:1 testcross (or backcross) ratio and signifies that one parent is doubly heterozygous, whereas the other is fully homozygous recessive. The answer is

$$WwGg \times wwgg$$

3-3. (a) When examining this cross

$$AaBbCc \times AaBBCC$$

expect there to be 8 different kinds of gametes from one parent (*AaBbCc*) and 2 different kinds from the other (*AaBBCC*). Therefore, there should be 16 kinds (genotypes) of offspring (8 × 2).

Gametes: Gametes:

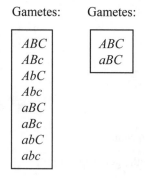

Offspring:

Genotypes	Ratio	Phenotypes
AABBCC	(1/16)	
AABBCc	(1/16)	
AABbCC	(1/16)	
AABbCc	(1/16)	
AaBBCC	(2/16)	$A\_B\_C\_ = 12/16$
AaBBCc	(2/16)	
AaBbCC	(2/16)	
AaBbCc	(2/16)	
aaBBCC	(1/16)	
aaBBCc	(1/16)	$aaB\_C\_ = 4/16$
aaBbCC	(1/16)	
aaBbCc	(1/16)	

(b) There will be four kinds of gametes for the first parent (*AaBBCc*) and two kinds of gametes for the second parent.

Gametes: Gametes:

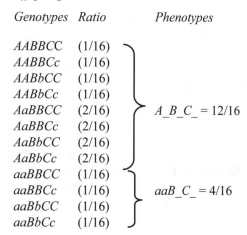

Offspring:

Genotypes	Ratio	Phenotypes
AaBBCC	1/8	$A\_BBC\_ = 3/8$
AaBBCc	2/8	

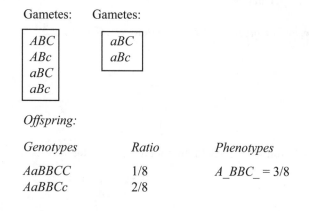

AaBBcc	1/8	*A_BBcc*	=1/8
aaBBCC	1/8	*aaBBC_*	= 3/8
aaBBCc	2/8		
aaBBcc	1/8	*aaBBcc*	= 1/8

(c) There will be eight (2^n) different kinds of gametes from each of the parents and therefore a 64-box Punnett square. Doing this problem by the forked-line method helps considerably.

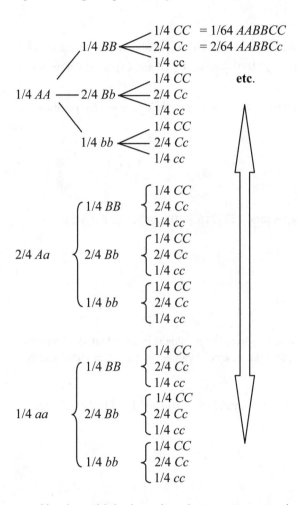

Simply multiply through each component to arrive at the final genotypic frequencies.

For the phenotypic frequencies, set up the problem in the following manner:

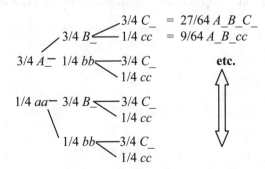

3-4. (a) One must think of this problem as a dihybrid F_2 situation with the following expectations:

Expected ratio	Observed (o)	Expected (e)
9/16	315	312.75
3/16	108	104.25
3/16	101	104.25
1/16	32	34.75

$$\chi^2 = 0.47$$

Looking at the table in the text, one can see that this χ^2 value is associated with a probability greater than 0.90 for 3 degrees of freedom (because there are now four classes in the χ^2 test). The observed and expected values do not deviate significantly.

To deal with parts **(b)** and **(c)**, it is easier to see the observed values for the monohybrid ratios if the phenotypes are listed:

smooth, yellow	315
smooth, green	108
wrinkled, yellow	101
wrinkled, green	32

For the smooth:wrinkled *monohybrid component*, the smooth types total 423 (315 + 108), whereas the wrinkled types total 133 (101 + 32).

Expected ratio	Observed (o)	Expected (e)
3/4	423	417
1/4	133	139

The χ^2 value is 0.35, and in examining the text for 1 degree of freedom, the *p* value is greater than 0.50 and less than 0.90. We fail to reject the null hypothesis and are confident that the observed values do not differ significantly from the expected values.

(c) For the yellow:green portion of the problem, there are 416 yellow plants (315 + 101) and 140 (108 + 32) green plants.

Expected ratio	Observed (o)	Expected (e)
3/4	416	417
1/4	140	139

The χ^2 value is 0.01, and in examining the text for 1 degree of freedom, the *p* value is greater than 0.90. We fail to reject the null hypothesis and are confident that the observed values do not differ significantly from the expected values.

Chapter 3 Mendelian Genetics

Solutions to Problems and Discussion Questions

1. (a) By noting that traits passed unaltered from parental to subsequent generations, Mendel not only postulated the "unit" or "particulate" nature of hereditary elements, but he also described their behavior. Results of various crosses provided the basis for knowing that factors can remain hidden in some circumstances, thereby implying two participating elements, one dominating the other. Predictable ratios in crosses supported the hypothesis of two hereditary elements involved in the expression of a given trait.

(b) Typically, by conducting a testcross, one readily tests whether an organism is homozygous or heterozygous for a given trait.

(c) In general, a chi-square analysis is used to compare observed data with various genetic models.

(d) Pedigree analysis is often used to determine whether and how traits are inherited in humans. However, other methods are also used and are discussed in subsequent chapters.

2. Several points surface in the first sentence of this question. First, two alternatives (black and white) of one characteristic (coat color) are being described; therefore, a monohybrid condition exists.

Second, are the guinea pigs in the parental generation (P₁) homozygous or heterozygous? Notice in the introductory sentence, just after PROBLEMS AND DISCUSSION QUESTIONS, there is the statement "members of the P_1 generation are homozygous F...."

Third, which is dominant, *black* or *white*? Note that all the offspring are black; therefore, black can be considered dominant. The second sentence of the problem verifies that a monohybrid cross is involved because of the 3/4 black and 1/4 white distribution in the offspring. Referring to appropriate text figures and knowing that genes occur in pairs in diploid organisms, one can write the genotypes and the phenotypes requested in part (a) as follows:

P_1:

Phenotypes:	Black	$\times$	White
Genotypes:	*WW*		*ww*
Gametes:			

F_1:   *Ww* (Black)

Ww	$\times$	*Ww*
¼ = *WW*		black
½ = *Ww*		black
¼ = *ww*		white

3. Start out with the following gene symbols:

A = normal (not albino),
a = albino.

Because albinism is inherited as a recessive trait, genotypes *AA* and *Aa* should produce the normal phenotype, whereas *aa* will give albinism. **(a)** The parents are both normal; therefore, they could be either *AA* or *Aa*. Because they produced an albino child, each parent must have provided an *a* allele to the albino child; thus, the parents must both be heterozygous (*Aa*). **(b)** To start out, the normal male could have either the *AA* or *Aa* genotype. The female must be *aa*. Because all the children are normal, one would consider the male to be *AA* instead of *Aa*. However, the male could be *Aa*. Under that circumstance, the likelihood of having six children, all normal, is 1/64.

4. Three of Mendel's postulates are illustrated in a problem such as this one. Unit factors occur in pairs (postulate 1) and demonstrate dominance/recessive relationships (postulate 2). The fact that these unit factors separate from each other during gamete formation illustrates postulate 3.

5. *Pisum sativum* is easy to cultivate and is naturally self-fertilizing, but it can be crossbred. It has numerous visible features (for example, tall or short, red flowers or white flowers) that are consistent under a variety of environmental conditions yet contrast due to genetic circumstances. Seeds could be obtained from local merchants. Three excellent books give insight into Mendel's life and the context of his discoveries: Carlson, E. A. 1966. *The Gene: A Critical History*. Philadelphia: W. B. Saunders; Sturtevant, A. H. 1965. *A History of Genetics*. New York: Harper and Row; Voeller, B. R. 1968. *The Chromosome Theory of Inheritance*. New York: Appleton-Century-Crofts.

6. In the first sentence, you are told that there are two *characteristics* that are being studied: seed shape and cotyledon color. Expect, therefore, this to be a

Chapter 3 Mendelian Genetics

dihybrid situation with *two gene pairs* involved. You can also see the possible alternatives of these two characteristics: *seed shape*, wrinkled vs. round; *cotyledon color*, green vs. yellow. After reading the second sentence, you can predict that the allele for round seeds is dominant to that for wrinkled seeds and the allele for yellow cotyledons is dominant to that for green cotyledons.

Symbolism:

w = wrinkled seeds   g = green cotyledons

W = round seeds   G = yellow cotyledons

P₁:

$$WWGG \times wwgg$$

Parents are considered to be homozygous for two reasons. First, in the introductory sentence, just after PROBLEMS AND DISCUSSION QUESTIONS, there is the statement "members of the P₁ generation are homozygous...." Second, notice that the only offspring are those with round seeds and yellow cotyledons.

Gametes produced: One member of each gene pair is "segregated" to each gamete.

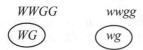

$$WWGG \qquad wwgg$$

F₁: WwGg

F₁ × F₁:

$$WwGg \times WwGg$$

Gametes produced: Under conditions of independent assortment, there will be four (2^n, where n = number of heterozygous gene pairs) different types of gametes produced by each parent.

Punnett square:

	WG	Wg	wG	wg
WG	WWGG	WWGg	WwGG	WwGg
Wg	WWGg	WWgg	WwGg	Wwgg
wG	WwGG	WwGg	wwGG	wwGg
wg	WwGg	Wwgg	wwGg	wwgg

Collecting the phenotypes according to the dominance scheme presented above gives the following:

9/16 W_G_ round seeds, yellow cotyledons
3/16 W_gg round seeds, green cotyledons
3/16 wwG_ wrinkled seeds, yellow cotyledons
1/16 wwgg wrinkled seeds, green cotyledons

Notice that an underscore (_) is used where, because of dominance, it makes no difference as to the dominant/recessive status of the allele.

Forked, or branch, diagram:

Seed shape	Cotyledon color	Phenotypes

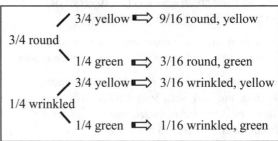

7. A testcross involves a cross of an organism with an unknown genotype to a fully homozygous recessive organism. In the problem Now Solve This 3-2, part **(c)** fits this description.

8. Because independent assortment may be defined as one gene pair segregating independently of another gene pair, one would need at least two gene pairs in order to demonstrate independent assortment. The problem satisfies criteria for Mendel's postulate of independent assortment.

9. Mendel's four postulates are related to the diagram below.

1. Factors occur in pairs. Notice A and a.
2. Some genes have dominant and recessive alleles. Notice A and a.
3. Alleles segregate from each other during gamete formation. When homologous chromosomes separate from each other at anaphase I, alleles will go to opposite poles of the meiotic apparatus.
4. One gene pair separates independently from other gene pairs. Different gene pairs on the same homologous pair of chromosomes (if far apart) or on nonhomologous chromosomes will separate independently from each other during meiosis.

28

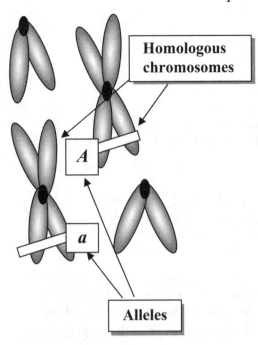

Homologous chromosomes

A

a

Alleles

10. Carefully reread the answer to question 3 in Chapter 2. Briefly, the factors that specify chromosomal homology are the following:

Overall length
Position of the centromere
Banding patterns
Type and location of genes
Autoradiographic pattern
Function

11. Homozygosity refers to a condition where both alleles of a gene pair are the same (for example, *AA* or *GG* or *hh*), whereas heterozygosity refers to the condition where members of a gene pair are different (for example, *Aa* or *Gg* or *Bb*). Homozygotes produce only one type of gamete, whereas heterozygotes will produce 2^n types of gametes, where *n* = number of heterozygous gene pairs (assuming independent assortment).

12. There are two characteristics presented here: body color and wing length. First, assign meaningful gene symbols.

Body color	Wing length
E = gray body color	*V* = long wings
e = ebony body color	*v* = vestigial wings

(a) P_1:

EEVV × *eevv*

F_1: *EeVv* (gray, long)

F_2: This will be the result of a Punnett square with 16 boxes, as in the text.

Phenotypes	Ratio	Genotypes	Ratio
gray, long	9/16	*EEVV*	1/16
		EEVv	2/16
		EeVV	2/16
		EeVv	4/16
gray, vestigial	3/16	*EEvv*	1/16
		Eevv	2/16
ebony, long	3/16	*eeVV*	1/16
		eeVv	2/16
ebony, vestigial	1/16	*eevv*	1/16

(b) P_1:

EEvv × *eeVV*

F_1: It is important to see that the results from this cross will be exactly the same as those in part **(a)** above. The only difference is that the recessive alleles are coming from both parents, rather than from one parent only as in **(a)**. The F_2 ratio will be the same as in **(a)** also. When you have genes on the autosomes (not X-linked), independent assortment, complete dominance, and no gene interaction (see later) in a cross involving double heterozygotes, the offspring ratio will be 9:3:3:1.

(c) P_1:

EEVV × *EEVv*

F_1: *EEVv* (gray, long)

F_2: Notice that all the offspring will have gray bodies, and you will get a 3:1 ratio of long to vestigial wings. You should see this before you even begin working through the problem. Even though this cross involves two gene pairs, it will give a monohybrid type of ratio because one of the gene pairs is homozygous (body color) and *one* gene pair is heterozygous (wing length).

Phenotypes	Ratio	Genotypes	Ratio
gray, long	3/4	*EEVV*	1/4
gray, vestigial	1/4	*EEvv*	1/4

Note: After working through this problem, it is important that you try to work similar problems without constructing the time-consuming Punnett squares, especially if each problem asks for phenotypic rather than genotypic ratios.

13. The general formula for determining the number of kinds of gametes produced by an organism is 2^n, where n = number of *heterozygous* gene pairs.

(a) 4: *AB, Ab, aB, ab*

(b) 2: *AB, aB*

(c) 8: *ABC, ABc, AbC, Abc, aBC, aBc, abC, abc*

(d) 2: *ABc, aBc*

(e) 4: *ABc, Abc, aBc, abc*

(f) $2^5 = 32$

14. In reading this question, notice that there are two characteristics being considered: seed color (yellow, green) and seed shape (round, wrinkled). At this point, you should be able to do this problem without writing down each of the steps. The F_1 can be considered to be a double heterozygote (with round and yellow being dominant). See the cross this way:

Symbols:

Seed shape	Seed color
W = round	*G* = yellow
w = wrinkled	*g* = green

P₁: *WWgg* × *wwGG*

F₁: *WwGg* cross to *wwgg*

(which is a typical testcross)

The offspring will occur in a typical 1:1:1:1 as

1/4 *WwGg* (round, yellow)

1/4 *Wwgg* (round, green)

1/4 *wwGg* (wrinkled, yellow)

1/4 *wwgg* (wrinkled, green)

Again, at this point, it would be very helpful if you could do such simple problems by inspection.

15. Because these are F_2 results from monohybrid crosses, a 3:1 ratio is expected for each. By referring to the text, one can set up the analysis easily.

(a)

Expected ratio	Observed (o)	Expected (e)
3/4	882	885.75
1/4	299	295.25

Expected values are derived by multiplying the expected ratio by the total number of organisms.

$$\chi^2 = \Sigma(o-e)^2/e = 0.064$$

In looking in the χ^2 table with 1 degree of freedom (because there were two classes, therefore, $n-1$ or 1 degree of freedom), we find a probability (p) value between 0.9 and 0.5.

We would therefore say that there is a "good fit" between the observed and expected values. Notice that as the deviations between the observed and expected values increase, the value of χ^2 increases. So the higher the χ^2 value, the more likely the null hypothesis will be rejected.

(b)

Expected ratio	Observed (o)	Expected (e)
3/4	705	696.75
1/4	224	232.25

$$\chi^2 = 0.39$$

The p value in the table for 1 degree of freedom is still between 0.9 and 0.5; however, because the χ^2 value is larger in (b), we should say that the deviations from expectation are greater. The deviation in each case can be attributed to chance.

16. It would be best to set up two tables based on the two hypotheses:

(a)

Expected ratio	Observed (o)	Expected (e)
3/4	250	300
1/4	150	100

(b)

Expected ratio	Observed (o)	Expected (e)
1/2	250	200
1/2	150	200

For the test of a 3:1 ratio, the χ^2 value is 33.3 with an associated *p* value of less than 0.01 for 1 degree of freedom. For the test of a 1:1 ratio, the χ^2 value is 25.0, again with an associated *p* value of less than 0.01 for 1 degree of freedom. Based on these probability values, both null hypotheses should be rejected.

17. Use of the *p* = 0.10 as the critical value for rejecting or failing to reject the null hypothesis instead of *p* = 0.05 would allow more null hypotheses to be rejected. Notice in the text that as the χ^2 values increase, there is a higher likelihood that the null hypothesis will be rejected because the higher values are more likely to be associated with a *p* value that is less than 0.05. As the critical *p* value is increased, it takes a smaller χ^2 value to cause rejection of the null hypothesis. It would take less difference between the expected and observed values to reject the null hypothesis; therefore, the stringency of failing to reject the null hypothesis is increased.

18. Given the cross $AaBbCC \times AABbCc$, we can apply the product rule, which states that when two or more events occur independently but simultaneously, their combined probability is equal to the product of their individual probabilities.

The probability of getting *AA* from

Aa × AA is 1/2

The probability of getting *Bb* from

Bb × Bb is 1/2

The probability of getting *Cc* from

CC × Cc is 1/2

The *overall* probability then is

1/2 × 1/2 × 1/2 = 1/8

19. The probability of getting *aabbcc* from the $AaBbCC \times AABbCc$ mating is zero because of homozygosity for *AA* and *CC*.

20. Although all the offspring will show the dominant A and C phenotypes and 3/4 will show the B phenotype, the probability of an offspring showing all three dominant traits would be $1 \times 3/4 \times 1 = 3/4$.

21. Although there are many different inheritance patterns that will be described later in the text (codominance, incomplete dominance, sex-linked

inheritance, etc.), the range of solutions to this question is limited to the concepts developed in the first three chapters, namely, dominance or recessiveness.

If an allele is dominant, it will not skip generations nor will it be passed to offspring unless at least one of the parents has the allele. On the other hand, alleles that are recessive can skip generations and exist in a carrier state in parents. For example, notice that II-4 and II-5 produce a female child (III-4) with the affected phenotype. On these criteria alone, the allele must be viewed as being recessive. Note: If an allele is recessive and X-linked (to be discussed later), the pattern will often be from affected male to carrier female to affected male.

To provide genotypes for each individual, consider that if the box or circle is shaded, the *aa* genotype is to be assigned. If offspring are affected (shaded), a recessive allele must have come from both parents.

I-1 (*Aa*), I-2 (*aa*), I-3 (*Aa*), I-4 (*Aa*)

II-1 (*aa*), II-2 (*Aa*), II-3 (*aa*), II-4 (*Aa*), II-5 (*Aa*), II-6 (*aa*), II-7 (*AA* or *Aa*), II-8 (*AA* or *Aa*)

III-1 (*AA* or *Aa*), III-2 (*AA* or *Aa*), III-3 (*AA* or *Aa*), III-4 (*aa*), III-5 (probably *AA*), III-6 (*aa*)

IV-1 through IV-7 (all *Aa*)

22. *Unit factors in pairs*: It is important to see that each time a phenotype (normal or abnormal) is stated, genotypes are symbolized as pairs of genes: *AA*, *Aa*, or *aa*. Review F3-2 to understand the need to assign appropriate symbols to genes.

Dominance and recessiveness: Because the gene for normal pigmentation is completely dominant over the gene for albinism (*a* is fully recessive), it was necessary to consider, at first, whether normally pigmented individuals in the problem were homozygous normal (*AA*) or heterozygous (*Aa*). By looking at the frequency of expression of the recessive gene in the offspring (in *aa* individuals), one can often distinguish an *Aa* type from an *AA* type.

Segregation: During gamete formation when homologous chromosomes move to opposite poles, paired elements (genes) separate from each other.

23. The allele is inherited as an autosomal recessive. Notice that two normal individuals II-3 and II-4 have produced a daughter (III-2) with myopia.

I-1 (*aa*), I-2 (*Aa* or *AA*), I-3 (*Aa*), I-4 (*Aa*)
II-1 (*Aa*), II-2 (*Aa*), II-3 (*Aa*), II-4 (*Aa*), II-5 (*aa*),
II-6 (*AA* or *Aa*), II-7 (*AA* or *Aa*)
III-1 (*AA* or *Aa*), III-2 (*aa*), III-3 (*AA* or *Aa*)

24. (a) There are two possibilities. Either the trait is dominant, in which case I-1 is heterozygous, as are II-2 and II-3, or the trait is recessive and I-1 is homozygous and I-2 is heterozygous. Under the condition of recessiveness, both II-1 and II-4 would be heterozygous, II-2 and II-3 homozygous.

(b) Recessive: Parents *Aa, Aa*

(c) Recessive: Parents *Aa, Aa*

(d) Recessive or dominant: if recessive, parents *AA* (probably), *aa*. Second pedigree: recessive or dominant, not sex-linked, if recessive, parents *Aa, aa*

25. (a) First consider that each parent is homozygous (true-breeding in the question), and because in the F_1, only round, axial, violet, and full phenotypes were expressed, they must each be dominant. Because all genes are on nonhomologous chromosomes, independent assortment will occur.

(b) Round, axial, violet, and full would be the most frequent phenotypes:

$$3/4 \quad \times \quad 3/4 \quad \times \quad 3/4 \quad \times \quad 3/4$$

(c) Wrinkled, terminal, white, and constricted would be the least frequent phenotypes:

$$1/4 \quad \times \quad 1/4 \quad \times \quad 1/4 \quad \times \quad 1/4$$

(d)

$$3/4 \quad \times \quad 3/4 \times \quad 3/4 \quad \times \quad 3/4 \quad +$$

$$1/4 \quad \times \quad 1/4 \quad \times \quad 1/4 \quad \times \quad 1/4 \quad = \quad 82/256$$

(e) There would be 16 different phenotypes in the testcross offspring just as there are 16 different phenotypes in the F_2 generation.

26. (a) Notice in cross #1 that the ratio of straight wings to curled wings is 3:1 and the ratio of short bristles to long bristles is also 3:1. This would indicate that straight is dominant to curled and short is dominant to long.

Possible symbols would be (using standard *Drosophila* symbolism):

straight wings = w^+ curled wings = w

short bristles = b^+ long bristles = b

(b)

Cross #1:	w^+/w ; b^+/b	$\times$	w^+/w ; b^+/b
Cross #2:	w^+/w ; b/b	$\times$	w^+/w ; b/b
Cross #3:	w/w ; b/b	$\times$	w^+/w ; b^+/b
Cross #4:	w^+/w^+ ; b^+/b	$\times$	w^+/w^+ ; b^+/b
	(one parent could be w^+/w)		
Cross #5:	w/w ; b^+/b	$\times$	w^+/w ; b^+/b

27. (a) First, consider that the data represent a 3:1 ratio based on the information given in the problem: $Ss \times Ss$. Compute the expected quantities for each class by multiplying the totals by 3/4 and 1/4.

Set I expected numbers:

Tall = 26.25
Short = 8.75

Set II expected numbers:

Tall = 262.5
Short = 87.5

For set I, the χ^2 value would be

$$(30 - 26.25)^2/26.25 \; + \; (5 - 8.75)^2/8.75$$

= 2.15, with p being between 0.2 and 0.05

so one would accept the null hypothesis of no significant difference between the expected and observed values.

For set II, the χ^2 value would be 21.43 and $p < 0.001$, and one would reject the null hypothesis and assume a significant difference between the observed and expected values.

(b) Clearly, with an increase in sample size, a different conclusion is reached. In fact, most statisticians recommend that the expected values in each class should not be less than 10. In most cases, more confidence is gained as the sample size increases; however, depending on the organism or experiment, there may be practical limits on sample size.

Chapter 4: Modification of Mendelian Ratios

Concept Areas	Corresponding Problems
Incomplete Dominance, Codominance	1, 2, 3, 5, 6, 7, 17, 24, 26
Multiple Alleles	4, 11, 26
Lethal Alleles	5
Gene Interaction	1, 18, 19, 22
Epistasis	8, 9, 20, 25
Complementation	23
X-Linkage	1, 10, 11, 13, 14, 15, 16, 21, 27, 32, 33
Sex-Limited, Sex-Influenced	12, 28
Extranuclear Inheritance	1, 29, 30, 31

Structures and Processes Checklist – Significant concepts that deserve special attention are identified with a "*".

(check topic when mastered – provide examples where appropriate – understand the context of each entry)

- **Modified Mendelian Ratios**
  - complex modes of inheritance*
  - gene interaction
  - various heritable patterns
- **Alleles Alter Phenotypes**
  - wild-type allele*
  - loss-of-function mutation*
  - null allele*
  - gain-of-function mutation*
  - neutral mutation*
- **Symbols for Alleles***
  - upper case/lower case
  - superscripts
  - *Drosophila*
  - italics
- nonitalics for gene products
- **Incomplete or Partial Dominance***
  - Tay-Sachs disease
  - hexoaminidase
- **Codominance***
  - MN blood group
  - both alleles expressed
- **Multiple Alleles***
  - number of alleles in population
  - ABO blood groups*
  - isoagglutinogen
  - Bombay phenotype
  - H substance
  - epistasis
  - fucosyl transferase

- **Lethal Alleles***
  - modified ratios
  - 2:1*
  - Huntington disease
- **Modified 9:3:3:1 Ratios***
- **Gene Interaction***
  - epigenesis
  - hereditary deafness
  - heterogeneous trait
  - epistasis*
  - hypostatic
  - recessive epistasis*
  - dominant epistasis*
  - 9:3:4*
  - 13:3:1
  - 9:7*
  - 9:6:1
  - 13:3
  - 10:3:3
  - 15:1*
  - 6:3:3:4
  - novel phenotypes*
- **Complementation Analysis***
  - same or different genes
  - complementation group
- **Multiple Effects of Single Gene***
  - pleiotropy*
  - Marfan syndrome
  - porphyria variegata

- **X-Linkage***
  - results of reciprocal crosses*
  - white eyes in *Drosophila*
  - crisscross pattern of inheritance*
  - chromosome theory of inheritance*
  - color blindness in humans
  - examples of X-linked traits*
- **Sex-Limited/Sex-Influenced***
  - genes not on X chromosome
  - hen-feathered*
  - pattern baldness*
- **Genetic Background and Environment***
  - penetrance*
  - expressivity*
  - genetic background*
  - position effects
  - temperature effects
  - conditional mutations*
  - temperature-sensitive mutations
  - permissive condition
  - restrictive condition
  - onset of genetic expression*
  - Tay-Sachs disease
  - Lesch-Nyhan syndrome
  - Duchenne muscular dystrophy
  - Huntington disease
  - genetic anticipation*

- o   myotonic dystrophy
- o   **Genomic (Parental) Imprinting***
    - o   gene silencing
    - o   Prader-Willi syndrome
    - o   Angelman syndrome
    - o   epigenesis*
    - o   DNA methylation
- o   **Extranuclear Inheritance***
    - o   organelle heredity*
    - o   heteroplasmy*
    - o   chloroplasts
- o   *Mirabilis jalapa*
- o   mitochondrial mutations*
- o   poky in *Neurospora*
- o   petite in *Saccharomyces*
- o   mitochondrial mutations in humans*
- o   MERRF
- o   LHON
- o   maternal effect*
- o   *Ephestia*
- o   *Drosophila* embryology*

T4-1 Examples of typical monohybrid and dihybrid ratios with several modifications.

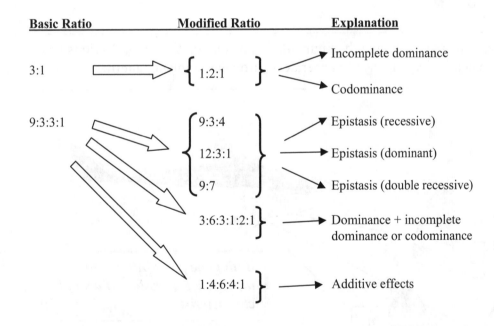

Basic Ratio	Modified Ratio	Explanation
3:1	1:2:1	Incomplete dominance
		Codominance
9:3:3:1	9:3:4	Epistasis (recessive)
	12:3:1	Epistasis (dominant)
	9:7	Epistasis (double recessive)
	3:6:3:1:2:1	Dominance + incomplete dominance or codominance
	1:4:6:4:1	Additive effects

F4-1 Illustration of gene interaction whereby products from more than one gene pair influence one characteristic or phenotypic trait.

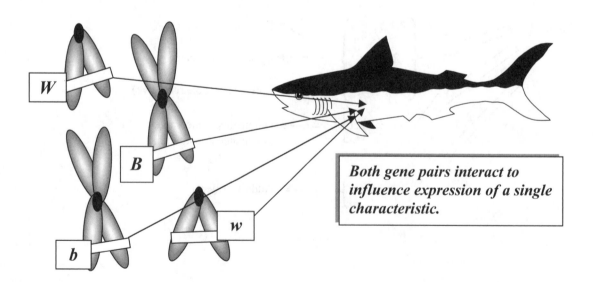

Arrangement of genes on chromosomes as viewed in metaphase chromosomes

B

A
A

a
a

b

One characteristic: gene interaction

Example: Two gene pairs influencing the pigmentation pattern on the shark. Various gene products contribute in a variety of ways to generate a particular pigment pattern.

W

B

b

w

Both gene pairs interact to influence expression of a single characteristic.

F4-2 Symbolism associated with the wild-type activity of a gene and several possible outcomes of the mutant state: **(A)** wild type, **(B)** too much product, **(C)** too little product, **(D)** no product, **(E)** both products expressed, **(F)** reduced product.

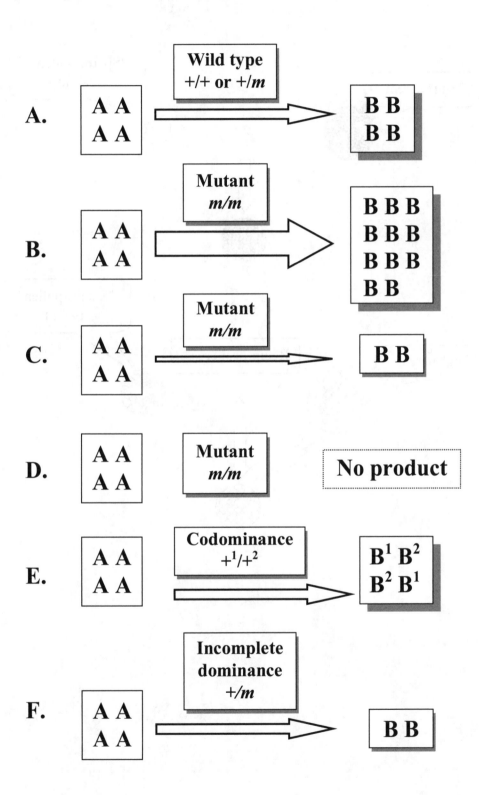

F4-3 Illustration of the common pattern seen in many cases of extranuclear inheritance. The condition of the female (egg) parent has a stronger influence on the phenotype of the offspring than that of the male (sperm/pollen) parent. Reciprocal crosses give different results in offspring.

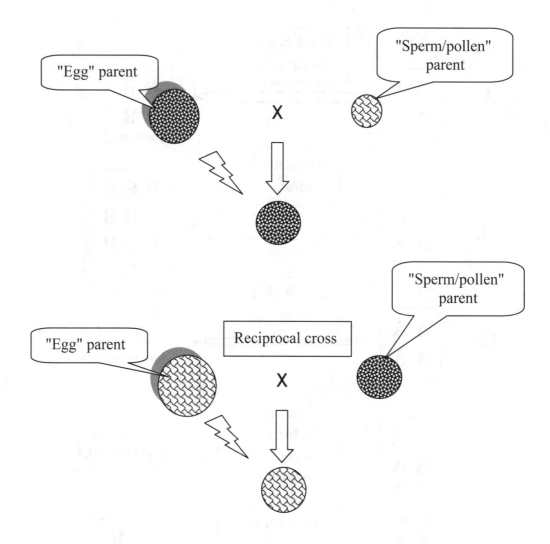

Answers to Now Solve This

4-1. It is important to see that this problem involves multiple alleles, meaning that monohybrid-type ratios are expected and that there is an order of dominance that will allow certain alleles to be "hidden" in various heterozygotes. As with most genetics problems, one must look at the phenotypes of the offspring to assess the genotypes of the parents.

(a)

Parents: sepia × cream

Because both guinea pigs had albino parents, both are heterozygous for the ca allele.

Cross: $c^k c^a$ × $c^d c^a$
2/4 sepia; 1/4 cream; 1/4 albino

(b)

Parents: sepia × cream

Because the sepia parent had an albino parent, it must be $c^k c^a$. Because the cream guinea pig had two sepia parents

$$(c^k c^d \times c^k c^d \quad \text{or} \quad c^k c^d \times c^k c^a)$$

the cream parent could be $c^d c^d$ or $c^d c^a$.

Crosses: $c^k c^a$ × $c^d c^d$
1/2 sepia; 1/2 cream*
*[if cream parent is homozygous]
or $c^k c^a$ × $c^d c^a$
1/2 sepia; 1/4 cream; 1/4 albino

(c)

Parents: sepia × cream

Because the sepia guinea pig had two full-color parents, which could be

$$Cc^k, \quad Cc^d, \quad \text{or} \quad Cc^a$$

(not *CC* because sepia could not be produced), its genotype could be

$$c^k c^k, \quad c^k c^d, \quad \text{or} \quad c^k c^a$$

Because the cream guinea pig had two sepia parents

$$(c^k c^d \quad \times \quad c^k c^d \quad \text{or} \quad c^k c^d \quad \times \quad c^k c^a)$$

the cream parent could be $c^d c^d$ or $c^d c^a$.

Crosses:

$c^k c^k \times c^d c^d \implies$ all sepia

$c^k c^k \times c^d c^a \implies$ all sepia

$c^k c^d \times c^d c^d \implies$ 1/2 sepia; 1/2 cream

$c^k c^d \times c^d c^a \implies$ 1/2 sepia; 1/2 cream

$c^k c^a \times c^d c^d \implies$ 1/2 sepia; 1/2 cream

$c^k c^a \times c^d c^a \implies$

1/2 sepia; 1/4 cream; 1/4 albino

(d)

Parents: sepia × cream

Because the sepia parent had a full-color parent and an albino parent ($Cc^k \times c^a c^a$), it must be $c^k c^a$. The cream parent had two full-color parents that could be Cc^d or Cc^a; therefore, it could be $c^d c^d$ or $c^d c^a$.

Crosses:

$c^k c^a \times c^d c^d \implies$ 1/2 sepia; 1/2 cream

$c^k c^a \times c^d c^a \implies$

1/2 sepia; 1/4 cream; 1/4 albino

4-2. Notice that the distribution of observed offspring fits a 9:3:4 ratio quite well. This suggests that two independently assorting gene pairs with epistasis are involved. Assign gene symbols in the usual manner:

A = pigment; a = pigmentless (colorless)

B = purple; b = red

$AaBb \times AaBb$
↓

$A\_B\_$	=	purple
A_bb	=	red
$aaB\_$	=	colorless
$aabb$	=	colorless

One may see this occurring in the following manner:

precursor ---+-> cyanidin ---+-> purple pigment

(colorless) *aa*   (red) *bb*

4-3. For all three pedigrees, let *a* represent the mutant gene and *A* represent its normal allele.

(a) This pedigree is consistent with an X-linked recessive trait because the male would contribute an X chromosome carrying the *a* mutation to the *aa* daughter. The mother would have to be heterozygous *Aa*.

(b) This pedigree is consistent with an X-linked recessive trait because the mother could be *Aa* and transmit her *a* allele to her one son (*a*/Y) and her *A* allele to her other son.

(c) This pedigree is not consistent with an X-linked mode of inheritance because the *aa* mother has an *A*/Y son.

Chapter 4 Modification of Mendelian Ratios

Solutions to Problems and Discussion Questions

1. (a) In general, they observed results of crosses that didnot produce offspring in typical Mendelian ratios.

(b) Modifications of dihybrid and higher-level ratios indicated that loci were not expressed independently. A 9:3:4 ratio illustrates such a dihybrid modification. The number of gene pairs involved is often determined by the sum of the components of each ratio. For example, a 1:2:1 or 3:1 ratio adds to four, indicating a monohybrid cross. A 9:3:4 or 15:1 ratio adds to 16, indicating a dihybrid ratio.

(c) Morgan and his colleagues observed that the sex of the parent carrying a mutant allele influenced the results of crosses when compared to a reciprocal cross. When correlated with the sex chromosome differences between males and females, a model placing a gene on the X chromosome was supported.

(d) When a gene is X-linked, ratios from crosses are influenced by which parent contributes a particular allele. When sex-limited or sex-influenced inheritance occurs, the parental source of the allele is irrelevant because the involved genes are autosomal.

(e) Scientists noted that in some cases, the pattern of inheritance did not follow what was expected of chromosomal genes. With organelle inheritance, the cytoplasm carried considerable influence on the phenotype of the mother, whereas in maternal effects, the genotype of the mother played a dominant role in determining the phenotype of the offspring.

2. In the first sentence of this problem, notice that there is one characteristic (coat color) and three phenotypes mentioned: red, white, and roan. The fact that roan is intermediate between red and white suggests that this may be a case of incomplete dominance, with roan being the intermediate and therefore the heterozygous type. If that is the case, then we should suspect a 1:2:1 phenotypic ratio in crosses of "roan to roan."

Looking at the data given, notice that a cross of the "extremes" (red × white) gives roan, suggesting its heterozygous nature and the homozygous nature of the parents. Seeing the 1:2:1 ratio in the offspring of

roan × roan

confirms the hypothesis of incomplete dominance as the mode of inheritance.

Symbolism:

AA = red

aa = white

Aa = roan

Crosses: It is important at this point that you not be fully dependent on writing out complete Punnett squares for each cross. Begin working these simple problems in your head.

AA × AA ⟹ AA

aa × aa ⟹ aa

AA × aa ⟹ Aa

Aa × Aa ↴

1/4 AA; 2/4 Aa; 1/4 aa

3. *Incomplete dominance* can be viewed as a quantitative phenomenon whereby the heterozygote is intermediate (approximately) between the limits set by the homozygotes. Pink is intermediate between red and white.

Codominance can be viewed in a more qualitative manner whereby both of the alleles in the heterozygote are expressed. For example, in the AB blood group, both the I^A and I^B genes are expressed. There is no intermediate class that is part I^A and I^B.

4. In this problem, remember that individuals with blood type B can have the genotype $I^B I^B$ or $I^B i^o$ and those with blood type A can have genotypes $I^A I^A$ or $I^A i^o$.

Male Parent: must be $I^B i^o$ because the mother is ii and one inherits one homolog (therefore one allele) from each parent.

Female Parent: must be $I^A i^o$ because the father is $I^B i^o$ and one inherits one homolog (therefore one allele) from each parent. The father can not be $I^B I^B$ and have a daughter of blood type A.

Offspring:

$I^A i^o$ × $I^B i^o$

	I^B	i^o
I^A	$I^A I^B$ (AB)	$I^A i^o$ (A)
i^o	$I^B i^o$ (B)	$i^o i^o$ (O)

The ratio would be

$$1(A):1(B):1(AB):1(O).$$

5. Notice that there is one typical (coat color) and one atypical (lethality) characteristic mentioned. Often under this condition of two characteristics, we must decide whether the problem involves one or more than one gene pair. Because the genotypes are given here, it is obvious that lethality is associated with expression of the coat color alleles and therefore one gene pair is involved. This is a monohybrid condition.

$Pp \times Pp$

1/4 PP (**lethal**)

2/4 Pp (platinum)

1/4 pp (silver)

Therefore, the ratio of surviving foxes is 2/3 platinum, 1/3 silver. The P allele behaves as a recessive in terms of lethality (seen only in the homozygote) but as a dominant in terms of coat color (seen in the homozygote).

6. Three independently assorting characteristics are being dealt with: flower color (incomplete dominance), flower shape (dominant/recessive), and plant height (dominant/recessive). Establish appropriate gene symbols:

Flower color:

RR = red; Rr = pink; rr = white

Flower shape:

P = personate; p = peloric

Plant height:

D = tall; d = dwarf

(a)

$RRPPDD \times rrppdd$

$RrPpDd$ (pink, personate, tall)

(b) Use *components* of the forked line method as follows:

2/4 pink $\times$ 3/4 personate $\times$ 3/4 tall

= 18/64

7. There are two characteristics: flower color and flower shape. Because pink results from a cross of red and white, one would conclude that flower color is monohybrid with incomplete dominance.

In addition, because personate is seen in the F_1 when personate and peloric are crossed, personate must be dominant to peloric. Results from crosses (c) and (d) verify these conclusions. The appropriate symbols would be as follows:

Flower color:

RR = red; Rr = pink; rr = white

Flower shape:

P = personate; p = peloric

(a)

$RRpp \times rrPP \implies RrPp$

(b)

$RRPP \times rrpp \implies RrPp$

(c)

$RrPp \times RRpp \implies$ $\begin{cases} RRPp \\ RRpp \\ RrPp \\ Rrpp \end{cases}$

(d)

$RrPp \times rrpp \implies$ $\begin{cases} rrPp \\ rrpp \\ RrPp \\ Rrpp \end{cases}$

In the cross of the F_1 of (a) to the F_1 of (b), both of which are double heterozygotes, one would expect the following:

$$RrPp \times RrPp$$

1/4 red — 3/4 personate → 3/16 red, personate

1/4 peloric → 1/16 red, peloric

2/4 pink — 3/4 personate → 6/16 pink, personate

1/4 peloric → 2/16 pink, peloric

1/4 white — 3/4 personate → 3/16 white, personate

1/4 peloric → 1/16 white, peloric

8. This is a case of gene interaction (novel phenotypes) whereby the yellow and black types (double mutants) interact to give the cream phenotype and epistasis whereby the cc genotype produces albino.

(a)

$AaBbCc \implies$ gray (C allows pigment)

(b)

$A\_B\_cc \implies$ albino

(c) Use the forked-line method for this portion.

$$3/4 A\_ \begin{cases} 3/4 B\_ \begin{cases} 1/2\ Cc \implies 9/32\ \text{gray} \\ 1/2\ cc \implies 9/32\ \text{albino} \end{cases} \\ 1/4\ bb \begin{cases} 1/2\ Cc \implies 3/32\ \text{yellow} \\ 1/2\ cc \implies 3/32\ \text{albino} \end{cases} \end{cases}$$

$$1/4\ aa \begin{cases} 3/4 B\_ \begin{cases} 1/2\ Cc \implies 3/32\ \text{black} \\ 1/2\ cc \implies 3/32\ \text{albino} \end{cases} \\ 1/4\ bb \begin{cases} 1/2\ Cc \implies 1/32\ \text{cream} \\ 1/2\ cc \implies 1/32\ \text{albino} \end{cases} \end{cases}$$

Combining the phenotypes gives (always count the proportions to see that they add up to 1.0):

16/32	albino
9/32	gray
3/32	yellow
3/32	black
1/32	cream

9. Treat each of the crosses as a series of monohybrid crosses, remembering that albino is epistatic to color and black and yellow interact to give cream.

(a) Because this is a 9:3:3:1 ratio with no albino phenotypes, the parents must each have been double heterozygotes and incapable of producing the cc genotype.

Genotypes:
  $AaBbCC \times AaBbCC$
      or
  $AaBbCC \times AaBbCc$
Phenotypes:
      gray $\times$ gray

(b) Because there are no black offspring, there are no combinations in the parents that can produce aa. The

4/16 proportion indicates that the C locus is heterozygous in both parents.

If the parents are

$AABbCc$	$\times$	$AaBbCc$
	or	
$AABbCc$	$\times$	$AABbCc$

then the results would follow the pattern given. Phenotypes: gray $\times$ gray.

(c) Notice that 16/64 or 1/4 of the offspring are albino; therefore, the parents are both heterozygous at the C locus. Second, notice that without considering the C locus, there is a 27:9:9:3 ratio that reduces to a 9:3:3:1 ratio. Given this information, the genotypes must be

$AaBbCc \times AaBbCc$

Phenotypes: gray $\times$ gray

10. In order to solve this problem, one must first see the possible genotypes of the parents and the grandfathers. Because the gene is X-linked, the cross will be symbolized with the X chromosomes.

RG = normal vision; rg = color-blind

Mother's father: X^{rg}/Y

Father's father: X^{rg}/Y

Mother: $X^{RG}X^{rg}$

Father: X^{RG}/Y

Notice that the mother must be heterozygous for the rg allele (being normal-visioned and having inherited an X^{rg} from her father) and the father, because he has normal vision, must be X^{RG}. The fact that the father's father is color-blind does not mean that the father will be color-blind. On the contrary, the father will inherit his X chromosome from his mother.

$$X^{RG} X^{rg} \times X^{RG}/Y$$

$X^{RG}X^{RG}$	=	1/4 daughter normal
$X^{RG}X^{rg}$	=	1/4 daughter normal
X^{RG}/Y	=	1/4 son normal
X^{rg}/Y	=	1/4 son color-blind

Looking at the distribution of offspring:

(a) 1/4

(b) 1/2

(c) 1/4

(d) zero

11. The mating is $X^{RG}X^{rg}$; $I^A i$ $\times$ $X^{RG}Y$; $I^A i$
Based on the son who is color-blind and blood type O, the mother must have been heterozygous for the *RG* locus and both parents must have had one copy of the I^O gene. The probability of having a female child is 1/2, that she has normal vision is 1 (because the father's X is normal), and that she has type O blood is 1/4. The final product of the independent probabilities is

$$1/2 \times 1 \times 1/4 = 1/8$$

12. Seeing the different distribution between males and females, one might consider sex-influenced inheritance as a model and have males more likely to express bearded and females more likely to express beardless in the heterozygote. This situation is similar to pattern baldness in humans. Consider two alleles that are autosomal and let

BB = beardless in both sexes
Bb = beardless in females
Bb = bearded in males
bb = bearded in both sexes

P_1: female: bb (bearded) × male: BB (beardless)

F_1: Bb = female beardless; males bearded

Because half of the offspring are males and half are females, one could, for clarity, rewrite the F_2 as:

	1/2 *females*	1/2 *males*
1/4 *BB*	1/8 beardless	1/8 beardless
2/4 *Bb*	2/8 beardless	2/8 bearded
1/4 *bb*	1/8 bearded	1/8 bearded

One could test the above model by crossing F_1 (heterozygous) beardless females with bearded (homozygous) males. Comparing these results with the reciprocal cross would support the model if the distributions of sexes with phenotypes were the same in both crosses.

13. The tortoiseshell condition is caused by the phenomenon of dosage compensation whereby one of the two X chromosomes is randomly inactivated in mammalian females. Once inactivated, all cells descending from a given cell will have the same X chromosome inactive. A tortoiseshell female is *Bb* and when crossed with a *BY* male produces the following offspring:

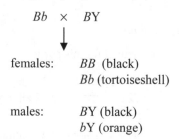

females: *BB* (black)
          Bb (tortoiseshell)

males: *BY* (black)
          bY (orange)

From the above information, it would seem impossible to get a tortoiseshell male; however, rare nondisjunction in the female can produce a tortoiseshell male with the *BbY* genotype.

14. Symbolism: Normal wing margins = sd^+; scalloped = sd

(a)

P_1: $X^{sd}X^{sd}$ × X^+/Y
F_1: 1/2 X^+X^{sd} (female, normal)
1/2 X^{sd}/Y (male, scalloped)
F_2: 1/4 X^+X^{sd} (female, normal)
1/4 $X^{sd}X^{sd}$ (female, scalloped)
1/4 X^+/Y (male, normal)
1/4 X^{sd}/Y (male, scalloped)

(b)

P_1: X^+/X^+ × X^{sd}/Y
F_1: 1/2 X^+X^{sd} (female, normal)
1/2 X^+/Y (male, normal)
F_2: 1/4 X^+X^+ (female, normal)
1/4 X^+X^{sd} (female, normal)
1/4 X^+/Y (male, normal)
1/4 X^{sd}/Y (male, scalloped)

If the *scalloped* gene were not X-linked, then all of the F_1 offspring would be wild-type (phenotypically) and a 3:1 ratio of normal to scalloped would occur in the F_2.

15. Assuming that the parents are homozygous, the crosses would be as follows. Notice that the X symbol may remain to remind us that the *sd* gene is on the X chromosome. It is extremely important to account for both the mutant genes and each of their wild-type alleles.

P₁: $X^{sd}X^{sd};\ e^+/e^+\ \times\ X^+/Y;\ e/e$

F₁:

   1/2 $X^+X^{sd};\ e^+/e$ (female, normal)

   1/2 $X^{sd}/Y;\ e^+/e$ (male, scalloped)

F₂:

	X^+e^+	X^+e	$X^{sd}e^+$	$X^{sd}e$
$X^{sd}e^+$				
$X^{sd}e$	Fill in box on your own.			
Ye^+				
Ye				

Phenotypes:

   3/16 normal female

   3/16 normal male

   1/16 ebony female

   1/16 ebony male

   3/16 scalloped female

   3/16 scalloped male

   1/16 scalloped, ebony female

   1/16 scalloped, ebony male

Forked-line method:

P₁: $X^{sd}X^{sd};\ e^+/e^+\ \times\ X^+/Y;\ e/e$

⇓

F₁: 1/2 $X^+X^{sd};\ e^+/e$ (female, normal)

   1/2 $X^{sd}/Y;\ e^+/e$ (male, scalloped)

F₂: Wings   Color

1/4	female, normal	⟨ 3/4 normal	3/16
		1/4 ebony	1/16
1/4	female, scalloped	⟨ 3/4 normal	3/16
		1/4 ebony	1/16
1/4	males, normal	⟨ 3/4 normal	3/16
		1/4 ebony	1/16
1/4	male, scalloped	⟨ 3/4 normal	3/16
		1/4 ebony	1/16

16. It is extremely important to account for both the mutant genes and each of their wild-type alleles.

(a)

P₁: $X^vX^v;\ +/+\ \times\ X^+/Y;\ b^r/b^r$

F₁:

   1/2 $X^+X^v;\ +/b^r$ (female, normal)

   1/2 $X^v/Y;\ +/b^r$ (male, vermilion)

F₂:

Eye color (X)   Eye color   (autosomal)

1/4	female, normal	⟨ 3/4 normal	3/16
		1/4 brown	1/16
1/4	female, vermilion	⟨ 3/4 normal	3/16
		1/4 brown	1/16
1/4	males, normal	⟨ 3/4 normal	3/16
		1/4 brown	1/16
1/4	male, vermilion	⟨ 3/4 normal	3/16
		1/4 brown	1/16

   3/16 = female, normal

   1/16 = female, brown eyes

   3/16 = female, vermilion eyes

   1/16 = female, white eyes

   3/16 = male, normal

   1/16 = male, brown eyes

   3/16 = male, vermilion eyes

   1/16 = male, white eyes

(b)

P₁: $X^+X^+;\ b^r/b^r\ \times\ X^v/Y;\ +/+$

F₁:

   1/2 $X^+X^v;\ +/b^r$ (female, normal)

   1/2 $X^+/Y;\ +/b^r$ (male, normal)

F₂:

Eye color (X)   Eye color (autosomal)

2/4	female, normal	⟨ 3/4 normal	
		1/4 brown	
1/4	male, normal	⟨ 3/4 normal	
		1/4 brown	
1/4	male, vermilion	⟨ 3/4 normal	
		1/4 brown	

6/16 = female, normal

2/16 = female, brown eyes

3/16 = male, normal

1/16 = male, brown eyes

3/16 = male, vermilion eyes

1/16 = male, white eyes

(c)

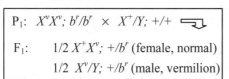

P_1: X^vX^v; b^r/b^r × X^+/Y; +/+

F_1: 1/2 X^+X^v; +/b^r (female, normal)
    1/2 X^v/Y; +/b^r (male, vermilion)

F_2:

Eye color (X)   Eye color (autosomal)

1/4 female, 3/4 normal
   normal 1/4 brown

1/4 female, 3/4 normal
   vermilion 1/4 brown

1/4 male, 3/4 normal
   normal 1/4 brown

1/4 male, 3/4 normal
   vermilion 1/4 brown

3/16 = female, normal

1/16 = female, brown eyes

3/16 = female, vermilion eyes

1/16 = female, white eyes

3/16 = male, normal

1/16 = male, brown eyes

3/16 = male, vermilion eyes

1/16 = male, white eyes

17. The key to dealing with this problem is seeing that there are two ways in which the sandy phenotype can be obtained. Notice that in cross 1, crossing sandy with sandy gives an F_1 with the all-red phenotype. Because the problem states that all the strains are true-breeding, there is likely some sort of complementation between the two sandy strains to give the all-red F_1 in cross 1. If you start out with that premise and assign the following genotypic possibilities, all the data fall into place:

A_B_ = red
A_bb or aaB_ = sandy
aabb = white

For the lost data in crosses 1 and 4, use the following:

Cross 1: aaBB × AAbb

  F_1: AaBb

  F_2:

  6/16 {
    9/16 = A_B_ (red)
    3/16 = A_bb (sandy)
    3/16 = aaB_ (sandy)
    1/16 = aabb (white)

Cross 4: aabb × AABB

  F_1: AaBb

  F_2:

  6/16 {
    9/16 = A_B_ (red)
    3/16 = A_bb (sandy)
    3/16 = aaB_ (sandy)
    1/16 = aabb (white)

18. (a) Because the denominator in the ratios is 64, one would begin to consider that there are three independently assorting gene pairs operating in this problem. Because there are only two characteristics (eye color and croaking), however, one might hypothesize that two gene pairs are involved in the inheritance of one trait, whereas one gene pair is involved in the other.

(b) Notice that there is a 48:16 (or 3:1) ratio of rib-it to knee-deep and a 36:16:12 (or 9:4:3) ratio of blue to green to purple eye color. Because of these relationships, one would conclude that croaking is due to one (dominant/recessive) gene pair, whereas eye color is due to two gene pairs. Because there is a 9:4:3 ratio regarding eye color, some gene interaction (epistasis) is indicated.

(c) Symbolism:

  Croaking: R_ = utterer; rr = mutterer

Eye color: Because the most frequent phenotype is blue eye, let A_B_ represent the genotypes. For the purple class, a 3/16 group uses the A_bb genotypes. The 4/16 class (green) would be the aaB_ and the aabb groups.

(d) The cross involving a blue-eyed, mutterer frog and a purple-eyed, utterer frog would have the genotypes

  AABBrr × AAbbRR

which would produce an F_1 of AABbRr, which would be blue-eyed and utterer. The F_2 would follow a pattern of a 9:3:3:1 ratio because of homozygosity for the A locus and heterozygosity for both the B and R loci.

9/16 *AAB_R_* = blue-eyed, utterer

3/16 *AAB_rr* = blue-eyed, mutterer

3/16 *AAbbR_* = purple-eyed, utterer

1/16 *AAbbrr* = purple-eyed, mutterer

19. In doing these types of problems, take each characteristic individually, then build the complete genotypes. Notice that the ratio of purple-eyed to green-eyed frogs is 3:1; therefore, expect the parents to be heterozygous for the *A* locus. Because the ratio of utterer to mutterer is also 3:1, expect both parents to be heterozygous at the *R* locus. The *B* locus would have the *bb* genotype because both parents are purple-eyed as given in the problem. Both parents would therefore be *AabbRr*.

20. Notice that in a cross between the F$_1$s in this problem, a 12:3:1 ratio is obtained, which is a clear sign that epistasis has modified a typical 9:3:3:1 ratio. In this case, cattle in one of the 3/16 classes have the same phenotype as cattle in the 9/16 class.

Because the 9/16 class typically takes the genotype of *A_B_*, it seems reasonable to think of the following genotypic classifications:

  *A_B_* = solid white (9/16)
  *aaB_* = solid white (3/16)
  A_bb = black and white spotted (3/16)
  aabb = solid black (1/16)

The selection of *bb* as giving the spotted phenotype is arbitrary. One could obtain *AAbb* true-breeding black and white spotted cattle.

21. (a, b) In looking at the pedigrees, one can see that the condition cannot be dominant because it appears in the offspring (II-3 and II-4) and not the parents in the first two cases. The condition is therefore *recessive*. In the second cross, note that the father is not shaded, yet the daughter (II-4) is. If the condition is recessive, then it must also be *autosomal*.

(c) II-1 = *AA* or *Aa*
  II-6 = *AA* or *Aa*
  II-9 = *Aa*

22. First, look for familiar ratios that will inform you as to the general mode of inheritance. Notice that the last cross (h) gives a 9:4:3 ratio, which is typical of epistasis. From this information, one can develop a model to account for the results given. Symbolism:

*A_B_* = black

A_bb = golden

aabb = golden

*aaB_* = brown

The combination of *bb* is epistatic to the *A* locus.

(a) *AAB_* × *aaBB* (other configurations are possible but each must give all offspring with *A* and *B* dominant alleles)

(b) *AaB_* × *aaBB* (other configurations are possible but both parents cannot be *Bb*)

(c) *AABb* × *aaBb*

(d) *AABB* × *aabb*

(e) *AaBb* × *Aabb*

(f) *AaBb* × *aabb*

(g) *aaBb* × *aaBb*

(h) *AaBb* × *AaBb*

Those genotypes that will breed true will be as follows:

  black = *AABB*

  golden = all genotypes that are *bb*

  brown = *aaBB*

23. The test for allelism is made by crossing the various mutant strains. If the resulting offspring are mutant, then the mutations are allelic. If the offspring are wild-type, then the mutations are not allelic and complementation is occurring. In cross 1, all the offspring are wild-type, indicating that *r1* and *r2* are complementing and therefore not allelic. In cross 2, all the offspring have tan eyes, indicating that the mutations are allelic. Because mutations *r1* and *r3* are in the same gene and *r1* and *r2* are not, the cross *r2* × *r3* should be complementing, that is, *r2* and *r3* are in different genes.

24. (a) This is a case of incomplete dominance in which, as shown in the third cross, the heterozygote (palomino) produces a typical 1:2:1 ratio. Therefore, one can set the following symbols:

  $C^{ch}C^{ch}$ = chestnut

  C^cC^c = cremello

  $C^{ch}C^c$ = palomino

(b) The F$_1$ resulting from matings between cremello and chestnut horses would be expected to be all palomino. The F_2 would be expected to fall in a 1:2:1 ratio as in the third cross in part (a) above.

25. This is a case in which epistasis (from *cc*) results in a "masking" of genes at the *A* locus. In this case, there will be modifications of typical 9:3:3:1 and 1:1:1:1 ratios because of gene interactions.

(a) In a cross of

$$AACC \ \times \ aacc$$

the offspring are all *AaCc* (agouti) because the *C* allele allows pigment to be deposited in the hair, and when it is, it will be agouti. F_2 offspring would have the following "simplified" genotypes with the corresponding phenotypes:

$A\_C\_$ = 9/16 (agouti)

A_cc = 3/16 (colorless because *cc* is epistatic to *A*)

$aaC\_$ = 3/16 (black)

$aacc$ = 1/16 (colorless because *cc* is epistatic to *aa*)

The two colorless classes are phenotypically indistinguishable; therefore, the final ratio is 9:3:4.

(b) Results of crosses of female agouti

$$(A\_C\_) \ \times \ aacc \text{ (males)}$$

are given in three groups:

(1) To produce an even number of agouti and colorless offspring, the female parent must have been *AACc* so that half of the offspring are able to deposit pigment because of *C*, and when they do, they are all agouti (having received only *A* from the female parent).

(2) To produce an even number of agouti and black offspring, the mother must have been *Aa*, and because no colorless offspring were produced, the female must have been *CC*. Her genotype must have been *AaCC*.

(3) Notice that half of the offspring are colorless; therefore, the female must have been *Cc*. Half of the pigmented offspring are black and half are agouti; therefore, the female must have been *Aa*. Overall, the *AaCc* genotype is likely.

26. First, make certain that you understand the genetics of all the gene pairs being described in the problem. The ABO system involves multiple alleles, codominance, and dominance. The MN system is codominant. The easiest way to approach these types of problems is to consider those gene pairs that produce a low number of options in the offspring. Notice in cross 1 that there are two options in the offspring for the ABO system (types A and O), but only one option for the MN system (type MN). By looking at the most restrictive classes, one can determine that option (c) is the only one that is both MN and O. The remainder of the combinations can be determined using the same logic.

$$\text{Cross } 1 \ = \ (c)$$
$$\text{Cross } 2 \ = \ (d)$$
$$\text{Cross } 3 \ = \ (b)$$
$$\text{Cross } 4 \ = \ (e)$$
$$\text{Cross } 5 \ = \ (a)$$

Given that each parental/offspring grouping can be used only once, there are no other combinations.

27. Passage of X-linked genes typically occurs from carrier mother to affected son. The fact that the father in couple 2 has hemophilia would not predispose his son to hemophilia. The first couple has no valid claim.

28. The clue to the solution comes from the description of the Dexters as not true-breeding and of low fertility. This indicates that the Dexters are heterozygous and the Kerry breed is homozygous recessive. The homozygous dominant type is lethal. Polled is caused by an independently assorting dominant allele, whereas horned is caused by the recessive allele to polled.

29. In cases of extranuclear inheritance, the phenotype is determined by the nuclear (maternal effect) or cytoplasmic (organelle or infectious) condition of the parent that contributes the bulk of the cytoplasm to the offspring. In most cases, the maternal parent provides the basis for the cytoplasmic inheritance.

The pattern of inheritance is more often from one parent to the offspring. One does not see both parents contributing to the characteristics of the offspring, as is the case with Mendelian (chromosomal) forms of inheritance. Standard Mendelian ratios (3:1) are usually not present. In general, the results of reciprocal crosses differ. See F4-3.

Female mutant × male wild

all offspring mutant

Female wild × male mutant

all offspring wild

In sex-linked inheritance, the pattern is often from grandfather through carrier mother to son. Patterns of extranuclear inheritance are often not influenced by the sex of the individual.

30. Developmental phenomena that occur early are more likely to be under maternal influence than those occurring late. Anterior/posterior and dorsal/ventral orientations are among the earliest to be established, and organisms whose study is experimentally and/or genetically approachable often show considerable maternal influence. Maternal effect genes produce products that are not carried over for more than one generation, as is the case with organelle and infectious heredity. Crosses that illustrate the transient nature of a maternal effect could include the following. (However, depending on particular biochemical/-developmental parameters, all crosses may not give these types of patterns.)

Female Aa × male aa -----> all offspring of the A phenotype.

Take a female A phenotype from the above cross and conduct the following mating: aa × male Aa. All offspring may be of the a phenotype because all of the offspring will reflect the *genotype* of the mother, not her *phenotype*. This cross illustrates that maternal effects last only one generation.

31. (a) The presence of bcd^-/bcd^- males can be explained by the maternal effect: mothers were bcd^+/bcd^-.

(b) The cross

female bcd^+/bcd^- Ξ male bcd^-/bcd^-

will produce an F_1 with normal embryogenesis because of the maternal effect. In the F_2, any cross having bcd^+/bcd^- mothers will have phenotypically normal embryos. Any cross involving homozygous bcd^-/bcd^- mothers will have problems with embryogenesis.

32. The mt^+ strain is the donor of the cpDNA because the inheritance of resistance or sensitivity is dependent on the status of the mt^+ gene.

33. Beatrice, Alice of Hesse, and Alice of Athlone are carriers. There is a 1/2 chance that Princess Irene is a carrier.

Chapter 5: Sex Determination and Sex Chromosomes

Concept Areas	Corresponding Problems
Sex Chromosomes	1, 2, 10, 11, 13, 14, 15, 17, 21, 26, 29
Nondisjunction	9, 14, 17
Life Cycles	3
Sex Determination	1, 4, 5, 6, 8, 25, 27, 28, 29
Sexual Differentiation	4, 12, 24, 25, 27, 28, 29
Dosage Compensation	1, 7, 16, 18, 19, 20, 21, 22, 23

Structures and Processes Checklist – Significant Concepts that deserve special attention are identified with a "∗".

(check topic when mastered – provide examples where appropriate – understand the context of each entry)

- **Sex Chromosomes∗**
  - heteromorphic
  - XY
  - sex determination
- **Life Cycles/Sexual Differentiation**
  - primary sexual differentiation∗
  - secondary differentiation∗
  - unisexual
  - dioecious∗
  - gonochroic
  - bisexual
  - monoecious∗
  - hermaphroditic
  - intersex
  - *Zea mays*
  - maize
  - sporophyte phase

- microspore
- microgametophyte
- megaspore mother cell
- pistil
- endosperm nuclei
- eight haploid nuclei
- antipodal nuclei
- pollination
- micropyle
- double fertilization∗
- *Caenorhabditis elegans*∗
- about 1000 cells
- males
- hermaphrodites
- X chromosome
- autosomes

Chapter 5 Sex Determination and Sex Chromosomes

- **X and Y Chromosomes***
  - heterochromosome
  - *Protenor* mode*
  - XX/XO
  - *Lygaeus turcicus**
  - XX/XY
  - heterogametic sex*
  - homogametic sex*
  - ZZ/ZW*
- **Y Chromosome***
  - Y determines maleness
  - 23 pairs in humans
  - Klinefelter syndrome (47, XXY)
  - Turner syndrome (45, X)
  - nondisjunction*
  - 47, XXX syndrome
  - triplo-X
  - 48, XXXX
  - 49, XXXXX
  - 47, XYY*
  - differentiation in humans*
  - gonadal (genital) ridges
  - cortex and medulla
  - bipotential gonads*
  - Y chromosome and maleness*
  - pseudoautosomal regions
  - PARs

- nonrecombining region of the Y
- NRY*
- male-specific region of the Y
- MSY*
- sex-determining region Y
- SRY*
- testis-determining factor
- TDF*
- transgenic mice
- *SOX9*
- **Ratio of Males to Females***
  - sex ratio*
  - primary sex ratio
  - secondary sex ratio
- **Dosage Compensation***
  - X-linked genes
  - Barr bodies
  - sex chromatin body
  - *N*-1 rule*
  - Lyon hypothesis*
  - tortoiseshell cats*
  - clone
  - G6PD*
  - mosaics
  - mechanism of inactivation*
  - imprinting*
  - epigenetics

- *Xic*
- *XIST*
- **Determination in *Drosophila****
  - XX/XY
  - nondisjunction studies*
  - contrary to humans*
  - metamales
  - intersexes

- genetic balance theory*
- X : A ratio*
- **Determinatin in Reptiles***
  - temperature-dependent*
  - ZZ/ZW
  - XX/XY
  - TSD
  - aromatase

Chapter 5 Sex Determination and Sex Chromosomes

Answers to Now Solve This

5-1. In mammals, the scheme of sex determination is dependent on the presence of a piece of the Y chromosome. If present, a male is produced. In *Bonellia viridis*, the female proboscis produces some substance that triggers a morphological, physiological, and behavioral developmental pattern that produces males. To elucidate the mechanism, one could attempt to isolate and characterize the active substance by testing different chemical fractions of the proboscis. Mutant analysis usually provides critical approaches to studying developmental processes. Depending on characteristics of the organism, one could attempt to isolate mutants that lead to changes in male or female development. By using micro-tissue transplantations, one could attempt to determine which anatomical "centers" of the embryo respond to the chemical cues of the female.

5-2. **(a)** Something is missing from the male-determining system of sex determination at the level of the genes, gene products, or receptors, and so on.

(b) The *SOX9* gene, or its product, is probably involved in male development. Perhaps it is activated by *SRY*.

(c) There is probably some evolutionary relationship between the *SOX9* gene and *SRY*. There is considerable evidence that many other genes and pseudogenes are also homologous to *SRY*.

(d) Normal female sexual development does not require the *SOX9* gene or gene product(s).

5-3. Because of X chromosome inactivation in mammals, scientists would be interested in determining whether the nucleus taken from Rainbow (donor) would continue to show such inactivation. Would the inactivated X chromosome retain the property of inactivation? The white patches of CC are due to an autosomal gene *S* for white spotting that prevents pigment formation in the cell lineages in which it is expressed. Homozygous *SS* cats have more white than heterozygous *Ss* cats, and there is no absolute pattern of patches due to the *S* allele. So the distribution of white patches would be expected to be different from Rainbow. In addition, because X chromosome inactivation is random, CC would have a different patch pattern from her genetic mother based on the random X inactivation basis alone.

Chapter 5 Sex Determination and Sex Chromosomes
Solutions to Problems and Discussion Questions

1. (a) Supported by the discovery of sex chromosome aneuploids (XO, XXY, for example), presence or absence of a Y chromosome has been shown to be fundamental in sex determination in humans.

(b) Based on consensus data of the sex of embryos and fetuses recovered from miscarriages and abortions, showing that fetal mortality is higher in males than females, it is estimated that the primary sex ratio favors males.

(c) The most direct evidence in support of random inactivation of either X chromosome in an XX cell came from experiments using electrophoretic variants of the G6PD locus. Such studies, coupled with mosaic coat patterns in mammals, support the random inactivation hypothesis.

(d) Calvin Bridges studied a number of chromosomal compositions in *Drosophila* and determined that the critical factor in sex determination is the ratio of X chromosomes to the number of haploid sets of autosomes. Given two haploid sets, XO is male and XXY is female.

2. The term *homomorphic* refers to the situation in which both the sex chromosomes have the same form. The term *heteromorphic* refers to the condition in many organisms when there are two different forms (morphs) of chromosomes such as X and Y. In *isogamous* species, there is little visible difference between the haploid vegetative cells that reproduce asexually and the haploid gametes that are involved in sexual reproduction. The two gametes that fuse during mating are morphologically indistinguishable and are called *isogametes*. An organism that is *heterogamous* is one in which there are two morphologically distinct sex chromosomes.

3. Maize (*Zea mays*) is a monoecious seed plant in which the sporophyte phase predominates during the life cycle. Both male and female structures are present on the adult plant. The stamens produce diploid microspore mother cells that undergo meiosis to produce four haploid microspores. Each haploid microspore develops into a microgametophyte that contains two sperm nuclei. Female diploid cells, megaspore mother cells, are located in the pistil of the sporophyte. Following meiosis, only one of the four haploid megaspores survives and divides mitotically three times, producing a total of eight

haploid nuclei. Two of these nuclei unite to become the endosperm nuclei. At the end of the sac where the sperm enters, three nuclei remain: the oocyte nucleus and two synergids. The other three antipodal nuclei cluster at the opposite end of the embryo sac.

When pollen grains make contact with the stigma and successfully develop, two sperm nuclei enter the embryo sac, one sperm nucleus unites with the haploid oocyte nucleus, and the other sperm nucleus unites with two endosperm nuclei.

Caenorhabditis elegans has two sexual phenotypes: males, which have only testes, and hermaphrodites, which contain both testes and ovaries. While in the larval stage of development of hermaphrodites, testes produce sperm, which are stored. Oogenesis does not occur until the adult stage is reached. The eggs are fertilized (self-fertilized) by the stored sperm. The majority of the offspring are hermaphrodites, whereas less than 1 percent of the offspring are males. As adults, males can mate with hermaphrodites, producing about half male and half hermaphrodite offspring.

4. Sexual differentiation is the response of cells, tissues, and organs to signals provided by the genetic mechanisms of sex determination. In other words, genes are present that signal developmental pathways whereby the sexes are generated. Sexual differentiation is the complex set of responses to those genetic signals.

5. The *Protenor* form of sex determination involves the XX/XO condition, while the *Lygaeus* mode involves the XX/XY condition.

6. In *Drosophila* it is the balance between the number of X chromosomes and the number of haploid sets of autosomes that determines sex. In humans there is a small region on the Y chromosome that determines maleness.

7. Mammals possess a system of X chromosome inactivation whereby one of the two X chromosomes in females becomes a chromatin body or Barr body. If one of the two X chromosomes is randomly inactivated, the dosage of genetic information is more or less equivalent in males (XY) and females (XX).

8. The Y chromosome is male determining in humans, and it is a particular region of the Y chromosome that causes maleness, the sex-determining region (SRY). SRY releases a product called the testis-determining factor (TDF), which causes the undifferentiated gonadal tissue to form testes. Individuals with the 47, XXY complement are males, while 45, XO produces females. In *Drosophila* it is the balance between the number of X chromosomes and the number of haploid sets of autosomes that determines sex. In contrast to humans, XO *Drosophila* are males and the XXY complement is female.

9. In *primary* nondisjunction, half of the gametes contain two X chromosomes while the complementary gametes contain no X chromosomes. Fertilization, by a Y-bearing sperm cell, of those female gametes with two X chromosomes would produce the XXY Klinefelter syndrome. Fertilization of the "no-X" female gamete with a normal X-bearing sperm will produce Turner syndrome.

10. (a) female $X^{rw}Y$ × male $X^{+}X^{+}$

F_1: females: $X^{+}Y$ (normal)
  males: $X^{rw}X^{+}$ (normal)

F_2: females: $X^{+}Y$ (normal)
    $X^{rw}Y$ (reduced wing)
  males: $X^{rw}X^{+}$ (normal)
    $X^{+}X^{+}$ (normal)

(b) female $X^{rw}X^{rw}$ × male $X^{+}Y$

F_1: females: $X^{rw}X^{+}$ (normal)
  males: $X^{rw}Y$ (reduced wing)

F_2: females: $X^{rw}X^{+}$ (normal)
    $X^{rw}X^{rw}$ (reduced wing)
  males: $X^{+}Y$ (normal)
    $X^{rw}Y$ (reduced wing)

11. No. Because the Y chromosome cannot be detected in these crosses, there is no way to distinguish the two modes of sex determination.

12. Males and females share a common placenta and therefore hormonal factors carried in blood. Hormones and other molecular species (transcription factors, perhaps) triggered by the presence of a Y chromosome lead to a cascade of developmental events that both suppress female organ development and enhance masculinization. Other mammals also exhibit a variety of similar effects depending on the sex of their uterine neighbors during development.

13. Because attached-X chromosomes have a mother-to-daughter inheritance and the father's X is transferred to the son, one would see daughters with the white eye phenotype and sons with the miniature wing phenotype. Attached-X plus X daughters would also be produced but would typically die as third-instar larvae. The YY combination is lethal to males.

14. If the male offspring had white eyes and the female offspring were wild-type, one might suspect that the attached-X had become unattached.

15. Because synapsis of chromosomes in meiotic tissue is often accompanied by crossing over, it would be detrimental to sex-determining mechanisms to have sex-determining loci on the Y chromosome transferred, through crossing over, to the X chromosome.

16. A *Barr body* is a differentially staining chromosome seen in some interphase nuclei of mammals with two X chromosomes. There will be one less Barr body than number of X chromosomes. The Barr body is an X chromosome that is considered to be genetically inactive.

17. There is a simple formula for determining the number of Barr bodies in a given cell: $N-1$, where N is the number of X chromosomes.

Klinefelter syndrome (XXY)	= 1
Turner syndrome (XO)	= 0
47, XYY	= 0
47, XXX	= 2
48, XXXX	= 3

18. The *Lyon hypothesis* states that the inactivation of the X chromosome occurs at random early in embryonic development. Such X chromosomes are in some way "marked" such that all clonally related cells have the same X chromosome inactivated.

19. Unless other markers, cytological or molecular, are available, one cannot test the Lyon hypothesis with homozygous X-linked genes. The test requires identification of allelic alternatives to see differences in X chromosome activity.

20. Females may display mosaic retinas with patches of defective color perception. Under these conditions, their color vision may be influenced.

21. Phenotypic mosaicism is dependent on the heterozygous condition of genes on the two X chromosomes. Dosage compensation and the formation of Barr bodies occur only when there are two or more X chromosomes. Males normally have only one X chromosome; therefore, such mosaicism cannot occur. Females normally have two X chromosomes. There are cases of male calico cats that are XXY.

22. Many organisms have evolved over millions of years under the fine balance of numerous gene products. Many genes required for normal cellular and organismic function in *both* males and females are located on the X chromosome. These gene products have nothing to do with sex determination or sex differentiation.

23. Like humans, *Drosophila* females contain two X chromosomes and males have only one X chromosome. Instead of X chromosome inactivation as seen in humans (mammals in general), male X-linked genes in *Drosophila* are transcribed at twice the rate as comparable genes on the X chromosome in *Drosophila* females.

24. There are several possibilities, which are discussed in the text. One could account for the significant departures from a 1:1 ratio of males to females by suggesting that at anaphase I of meiosis, the Y chromosome more often goes to the pole that produces the more viable sperm cells. One could also speculate that the Y-bearing sperm has a higher likelihood of surviving in the female reproductive tract, or that the egg surface is more receptive to Y-bearing sperm. At this time, the mechanism is unclear. As Pergament et al. (2002) Reprod Biomed Online July-Aug (5)(1) 43–46 explain:

"A number of environmental, physiological and genetic factors have been observed to impact on the primary sex ratio: sexual behaviour, variation in hormonal concentrations, natural disasters, environmental pollutants and timing of conception. Nevertheless, no biological mechanism or interaction of factors has suitably explained this phenomenon, or that of the prenatal vulnerability of the male, the suspected higher sex ratio in spontaneous abortion and the male excesses in adult diseases related to the intrauterine environment."

25. Because there is a region of synapsis close to the *Sry*-containing section on the Y chromosome, crossing over in this region would generate XY translocations that would lead to the condition described.

26. Because of the homology between the *red* and *green* genes, the possibility exists for an irregular synapsis (see the figure below) that, following crossing over, would give a chromosome with only one (*green*) of the duplicated genes. When this X chromosome combines with the normal Y chromosome, the son's phenotype can be explained.

Normal synapsis:

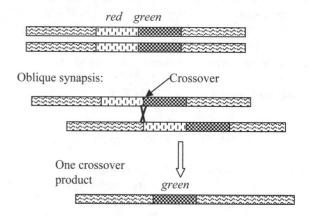

27. The presence of the Y chromosome provides a factor (or factors) that leads to the initial specification of maleness. Subsequent expression of secondary sex characteristics must be dependent on the interaction of the normal X-linked *Tfm* allele with testosterone. Without such interaction, differentiation takes the female path.

28. In snapping turtles, sex determination is strongly influenced by temperature such that males are favored in the 26–34°C range. Lizards, on the other hand, appear to have their sex determined by factors other than temperature in the 20–40°C range.

29. In human males, one copy of the SRY gene provides for testis development, whereas in chickens, two copies of *DMRT1* are required. The general architecture of sex determination in fowl is comparable to that in humans; however, it is somewhat reversed: females being the heterogametic sex, but the sex-determining genes function on the homogametic chromosomes of the male.

Chapter 6: Chromosome Mutations: Variation in Number and Arrangement

Concept Areas	Corresponding Problems
Variation in Chromosome Number	1, 2, 3, 4, 5, 6, 7, 8, 13, 14, 15, 16, 17, 18
Nondisjunction	1, 3, 5, 23, 25
Deletions	3, 9
Duplications	1, 3, 9, 12
Inversions	3, 10, 11, 19
Translocations	3, 20, 21, 22, 24, 26

Structures and Processes Checklist – Significant concepts that deserve special attention are identified with a "*".

(check topic when mastered – provide examples where appropriate – understand the context of each entry)

- **Chromosome Mutations***
  - aberrations
- **Variation in Number***
  - aneuploid/euploid*
  - Klinefelter syndrome
  - Turner syndrome
  - nondisjunction*
  - XXY
  - XO
- **Monosomy and Trisomy***
  - haploin sufficiency
  - 2*n* – 1
  - 2*n* + 1
  - Down syndrome
  - trisomy 21
  - Down syndrome critical region
  - DSCR

- *DSCR1*
- *VEGF*
- angiogenesis
- nondisjunction in meiosis*
- mostly in meiosis I
- maternal preference
- maternal age*
- amniocentesis
- chorionic villus sampling
- NIPGD
- Patau syndrome
- Edwards syndrome
- 47, 13+
- 47, 18+
- **Polyploidy***
  - autopolyploidy*
  - allopolyploidy*

- ○ amphidiploids*
- ○ American cotton
- ○ wheat
- ○ rye
- ○ autotriploids*
- ○ autotetraploids*
- ○ commercial applications
- ○ seedless plants
- ○ G1 cyclins*
- ○ cell size increase
- ○ **Composition and Arrangement***
  - ○ deletion*
  - ○ deficiency
  - ○ terminal
  - ○ intercalary
  - ○ compensation loop*
  - ○ cri du chat syndrome
  - ○ segmental deletion
  - ○ *TERT*
- ○ **Duplication***
  - ○ gene amplification
  - ○ ribosomal RNA genes
  - ○ rDNA
  - ○ nucleolar organizer region

- ○ NOR
- ○ *Bar* mutation
- ○ duplications in evolution*
- ○ trypsin, chymotrypsin
- ○ myoglobin
- ○ hemoglobin
- ○ **Inversions***
  - ○ paracentric*
  - ○ pericentric*
  - ○ sticky ends
  - ○ inversion heterozygotes*
  - ○ inversion loop*
  - ○ evolutionary advantages*
  - ○ balancer chromosomes
- ○ **Translocations***
  - ○ semisterility*
  - ○ familial Down syndrome
  - ○ Robertsonian translocation
- ○ **Fragile Sites***
  - ○ fragile-X syndrome
  - ○ Martin-Bell syndrome
  - ○ trinucleotide repeats*
  - ○ genetic anticipation*
  - ○ fragile sites and cancer

F6-1 Illustration of the chromosomal configurations of diploid and euploid genomes of *Drosophila melanogaster*.

Drosophila melanogaster female

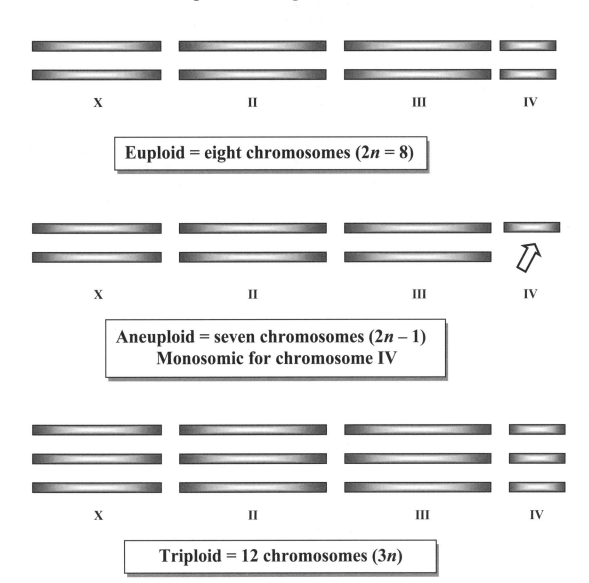

X   II   III   IV

Euploid = eight chromosomes (2*n* = 8)

X   II   III   IV

Aneuploid = seven chromosomes (2*n* – 1)
Monosomic for chromosome IV

X   II   III   IV

Triploid = 12 chromosomes (3*n*)

Answers to Now Solve This

6-1. A Turner syndrome female has the sex chromosome composition of XO. If the father had hemophilia, it is likely that the Turner syndrome individual inherited the X chromosome from the father and no sex chromosome from the mother. If nondisjunction occurred in the mother, either during meiosis I or meiosis II, an egg with no X chromosome can be the result. See the text for a diagram of primary and secondary nondisjunction.

6-2. The sterility of interspecific hybrids is often caused by a high proportion of univalents in meiosis I. As such, viable gametes are rare and the likelihood of two such gametes "meeting" is remote. Even if partial homology of chromosomes allows some pairing, sterility is usually the rule. The horticulturist may attempt to reverse the sterility by treating the sterile hybrid with colchicine. Such a treatment, if successful, may double the chromosome number, so each chromosome would now have a homolog with which to pair during meiosis.

6-3. The rare double crossovers within the boundaries of a paracentric inversion heterozygote produce only minor departures from the standard chromosomal arrangement as long as the crossovers involve the same two chromatids. With two-strand double crossovers, the second crossover negates the first. However, three-strand and four-strand double crossovers have consequences that lead to anaphase bridges as well as a high degree of genetically unbalanced gametes.

Chapter 6 Chromosome Mutations: Variation in Number and Arrangement

Solutions to Problems and Discussion Questions

1. (a) Before the advent of polymorphic markers, maternal involvement in trisomy 21 was strongly suspected because of the striking influence of maternal age on incidence. **(b)** Karyotype analysis of spontaneously aborted fetuses has shown that a significant percentage of abortuses are trisomic and every chromosome can be involved. Other forms of aneuploidy (monosomy, nullisomy) are less represented. **(c)** A variety of studies, many tracing to early work with specialized (polytene) chromosomes in *Drosophila* and aneuploidy in other organisms, demonstrated that as chromosome structures or numbers are altered, phenotypic consequences are likely. **(d)** By examining the polytene chromosomes of *Drosophila*, Bridges and Muller determined that the Bar-eye phenotype was caused by a chromosomal duplication of the 16A region on the X chromosome. In addition, unequal crossing over that resulted in reduced or increased numbers of 16A regions reverted or enhanced the Bar-eye phenotype.

2. With a diploid chromosome number of 18 (2*n*), a haploid (*n*) would have nine chromosomes, a triploid (3*n*) would have 27 chromosomes, and a tetraploid (4*n*) would have 36 chromosomes. A trisomic would have one extra chromosome (19) and a monosomic one less than the diploid (17).

3. With frequent exceptions, especially in plants, organisms typically inherit one chromosome complement (*haploid* = *n* = one representative of each chromosome) from each parent. Such organisms are *diploid*, or 2*n*. When an organism contains complete multiples of the *n* complement (3*n*, 4*n*, 5*n*, etc.), it is said to be *euploid,* in contrast to aneuploid, in which complete haploid sets do not occur. An example of an aneuploid is *trisomy,* whereby a chromosome is added to the 2*n* complement. In humans, trisomy 21 would be symbolized as 2*n* + 1 or 47, 21+.

Monosomy is an aneuploid condition in which one member of a chromosome pair is missing, thus producing the chromosomal formula of 2*n* – 1. Haplo-IV is an example of monosomy in *Drosophila*. *Trisomy* is the chromosomal condition of 2*n* + 1, whereby an extra chromosome is present. Down syndrome is an example in humans (47, 21+). See the text and notice that all the chromosomes are present in the diploid state except chromosome 21.

Patau syndrome is a chromosomal condition in which there is an extra D group chromosome. Such individuals are 47, 13+ and have multiple congenital malformations. *Edwards syndrome* is a chromosomal condition in which there is an extra E group chromosome (47, 18+). Individuals with Edwards syndrome have multiple congenital malformations and reduced life expectancy.

Polyploidy refers to instances when there are more than two haploid sets of chromosomes in an individual cell. *Autopolyploidy* refers to cases of polyploidy in which the chromosomes in the individual originate from the same species.

Allopolyploidy involves instances when the chromosomes originate from the hybridization of two different species, usually closely related.

Pericentric inversions have breakpoints that include the centromere, whereas *paracentric* inversions have breakpoints that do not include the centromere.

4. Individuals with Down syndrome, although suffering congenital defects, tendencies toward respiratory disease, and leukemia, can live well into adulthood. Individuals with Patau or Edwards syndrome live less than four months on the average. Comparing the different sizes of the involved chromosomes (21, 13, and 18, respectively), for example, suggests that the larger the chromosome, the lower the likelihood of lengthy survival. In addition, it would be expected that certain chromosomes, because of their genetic content, may have different influences on development.

5. Primary oocytes are formed by birth in females, and it isn't until ovulation and fertilization that meiosis is completed. Because progression of meiosis is not continuous, it has been suggested that the long period of chromosomal synapsis and recombination may be involved in the nondisjunctional process in females.

6. Because an allotetraploid has a possibility of producing bivalents at meiosis I, it would be considered the most fertile of the three. Having an even number of chromosomes to match up at the metaphase I plate, autotetraploids would be considered more fertile than autotriploids.

7. Early development is dependent on a synchronous interplay of numerous pulses of gene activity coordinated in time and space. Diploid organisms have evolved under the influence of two copies of each gene (except for sex chromosome involvement). When a chromosome is missing, the diploid state is not achieved and the genetic balance necessary for normal development fails early.

8. American cultivated cotton has 26 pairs of chromosomes: 13 large, 13 small. Old World cotton has 13 pairs of large chromosomes, and American wild cotton has 13 pairs of small chromosomes. It is likely that an interspecific hybridization occurred followed by chromosome doubling. These events probably produced a fertile amphidiploid (allotetraploid). Experiments have been conducted to reconstruct the origin of American cultivated cotton.

9. Basically, the synaptic configurations produced by chromosomes bearing a deletion or duplication (on one homolog) are very similar. There will be point-for-point pairing in all sections that are capable of pairing. The section that has no homolog will "loop out," as shown in the text.

10. Although there is the appearance that crossing over is suppressed in inversion heterozygotes, the phenomenon extends from the fact that the crossover chromatids end up being abnormal in genetic content. As such, they fail to produce viable (or competitive) gametes or lead to zygotic or embryonic death. Notice in the text that the crossover chromatids end up genetically unbalanced.

11. Crossing over in the inversion loop of a pericentric heterozygote produces all chromatids with centromeres, but the two chromatids involved in the crossover are genetically unbalanced. The balanced chromatids are of either normal or inverted sequence.

12. Modern globin genes resulted from a duplication event in an ancestral gene about 500 million years ago. Mutations occurred over time, and a chromosomal aberration separated the duplicated genes, leaving the eventual α cluster on chromosome 16 and the eventual β cluster on chromosome 11. In a work entitled *Evolution by Gene Duplication*, Ohno suggests that gene duplication has been essential in the origin of new genes. If gene products serve essential functions, mutation, and therefore evolution, would not be possible unless these gene products

could be compensated by products of duplicated, normal genes. The duplicated genes, or the original genes themselves, would be able to undergo mutational "experimentation" without necessarily threatening the survival of the organism.

13. The primrose, *Primula kewensis*, with its 36 chromosomes, is likely to have formed from the hybridization and subsequent chromosome doubling of a cross between the two other species, each with 18 chromosomes. An example of this type of allotetraploidy (amphidiploidy) is seen in the text.

14. Given the basic chromosome set of nine unique chromosomes (a haploid complement), other forms with the "*n* multiples" are forms of autotetraploidy. In the illustration below the *n* basic set is multiplied to various levels as is the autotetraploid in the example.

Basic set of nine unique chromosomes (*n*)

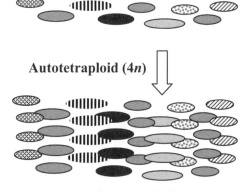

Autotetraploid (4*n*)

Individual organisms with 27 chromosomes are triploids (3*n*) and are more likely to be sterile because there are trivalents at meiosis I that cause a relatively high number of unbalanced gametes to be formed.

15. Set up the cross in the usual manner, realizing that recessive genes in the Haplo-IV individual will be expressed.

Let b = bent bristles; b^+ = normal bristles.

(a)

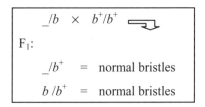

F₂:

$\_/b^+ \times b/b^+$ ⤵

$\_/b^+$	=	normal bristles
$\_/b$	=	bent bristles
b^+/b^+	=	normal bristles
b/b^+	=	normal bristles

(b)

$\_/b^+ \times b/b$ ⤵

F₁:

$\_/b$	=	bent bristles
b/b^+	=	normal bristles

F₂:

$\_/b \times b/b^+$ ⤵

$\_/b^+$	=	normal bristles
$\_/b$	=	bent bristles
b^+/b	=	normal bristles
b/b	=	bent bristles

16. The cross would be as follows:

$WWWW \times wwww$

(assuming that chromosomes pair at meiosis)

F₁: $WWww$

F₂:　　　　$1WW$　　　$4Ww$　　　$1ww$

$1WW$	
$4Ww$	$35W\_\_\_$ and $1wwww$
$1ww$	

17. Given some of the information in the preceding problem, the expression would be as follows:

$(35/36W\_\_\_:1/36wwww) \times$
$(35/36A\_\_\_:1/36aaaa)$ ⤵

$(35/36)^2$	$W\_\_\_A\_\_\_$
$35/(36)^2$	$W\_\_\_aaaa$
$35/(36)^2$	$wwwwA\_\_\_$
$1/(36)^2$	$wwwwaaaa$

18. Because two Gl_1 alleles and two ws_3 alleles are present in the triploid, they must have come from the pollen parent. The wording of the problem implies that the pollen parent contributed an unreduced ($2n$) gamete; however, another explanation, dispermic fertilization, is possible. In this case, two Gl_1ws_3 gametes could have fertilized the ovule.

19. (a) In all probability, crossing over in the inversion loop of an inversion (in the heterozygous state) produced defective, unbalanced chromatids, thus leading to stillbirths and/or malformed children.

(b) It is probable that a significant proportion (perhaps 50 percent if there is a high frequency of crossing over in the inversion) of the children of the man will be similarly influenced by the inversion.

(c) Because the karyotypic abnormality is observable, it may be possible to detect some of the abnormal chromosomes of the fetus by amniocentesis or CVS. However, depending on the type of inversion and the ability to detect minor changes in banding patterns, not all abnormal chromosomes may be detected.

20. (a) reciprocal translocation

(b)

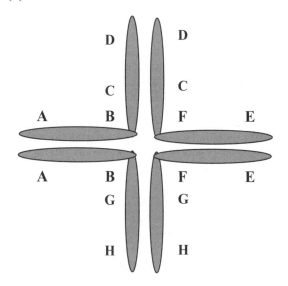

(c) Notice that all chromosomal segments are present and there is no apparent loss of chromosomal material. However, if the breakpoints for the translocation occurred within genes, then an abnormal phenotype may be the result. In addition, a gene's function is sometimes influenced by its position—its neighboring genes, in other words. If such "position effects" occur, then a different phenotype may result.

21. (a, b, c) It is likely that the translocation described above is the cause of the miscarriages. Segregation of the chromosomal elements will produce approximately half unbalanced gametes. The chance of a normal child is approximately one in two; however, half of the normal children will be translocation carriers. Should she abandon her attempts to have a child of her own?

The answer to this question is one more of personal choice than science. It is the task of the scientific community to provide accurate information within the limits of technology. Generally speaking, this information is provided to individuals so that they can make informed decisions. In this case, the woman has been given information that probably fits her circumstance. It is up to her to make such a personal decision.

22. The symbol t(14;21) indicates that part of chromosome 21 is translocated to chromosome 14. When a gamete containing such a chromosome plus a normal chromosome 21 is fertilized by a standard haploid gamete, the individual has 46 chromosomes but effectively has three copies of chromosome 21.

23. (a) The father must have contributed the abnormal X-linked gene.

(b) Because the son is XXY and heterozygous for anhidrotic dysplasia, he must have received both the defective gene and the Y chromosome from his father. Thus, nondisjunction must have occurred during meiosis I.

(c) This son's mosaic phenotype is caused by X chromosome inactivation, a form of dosage compensation in mammals.

24. First consider what is meant by a Robertsonian translocation: breaks at the short arms of two nonhomologous acrocentric chromosomes where the small acentric fragments are lost and the larger chromosomal segments fuse at or near the centromeric region, producing a compound, larger submetacentric or metacentric chromosome. Below is a description of breakage/reunion events that illustrate such a translocation in the relatively small, similarly sized chromosomes 19 (metacentric) and 20 (metacentric/submetacentric). The case described here is shown occurring before S phase duplication. The same phenomenon is shown in the text as

occurring after S phase. Because the likelihood of such a translocation is fairly small in a general population, inbreeding played a significant role in allowing the translocation to "meet itself."

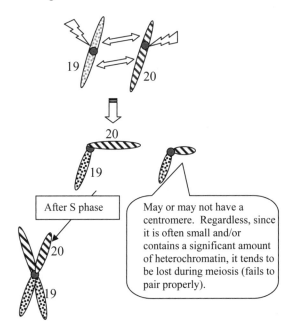

25. It is likely that mitotic nondisjunction contributed to the mosaic condition. If one of the X chromosomes failed to be included in a daughter mitotic cleavage cell, then a substantial proportion of the child's cells would be XO. Expression of Turner syndrome characteristics would depend on the percentage and location of the XO cell population. Mosaicism can also be caused by embryonic fusion, twin embryos fusing together to form one individual. If one embryo is XX and the other XO, the mosaicism could be explained.

26. This female will produce meiotic products of the following types:

normal: 18 + 21
translocated: 18/21
translocated plus 21: 18/21 + 21
deficient: 18 only

Note: The 18/21 + 18 gamete is not formed because it would require separation of primarily homologous chromosomes at anaphase I.

Fertilization with a normal 18 + 21 sperm cell will produce the following offspring:

normal: 46 chromosomes
translocation carrier: 45 chromosomes 18/21 + 18 + 21
trisomy 21: 46 chromosomes 18/21 + 21 + 21
monosomic: 45 chromosomes 18 + 18 + 21, lethal

Chapter 7: Linkage and Chromosome Mapping in Eukaryotes

Concept Areas	Corresponding Problems
Linkage vs. Independent Assortment	1, 21, 22, 23
Gene Mapping	1, 4, 8, 9, 10, 11, 12, 20, 24
Multiple Crossovers	3, 13, 14, 15, 16, 17, 18, 19
Determining Gene Sequence	14, 15, 16, 19
Interference and Coefficient of Coincidence	7, 14
Crossing Over in the Four-Strand Stage	1, 5
Mechanism of Crossing Over	1, 3, 4, 6, 25, 28
Human Maps	26, 27
Evolutionary Aspects	2

Structures and Processes Checklist – Significant concepts that deserve special attention are identified with a "*".

(check topic when mastered – provide examples where appropriate – understand the context of each entry)

- **Linkage and Recombination***
  - independent assortment*
  - parental gametes*
  - noncrossover gametes*
  - recombinant gametes*
  - crossover gametes*
  - 50 percent maximum*
  - linkage ratio
  - linkage group*
- **Gene Mapping***
  - Morgan, Sturtevant
  - chiasma
  - recombinant gametes
  - parental gametes
  - crossing over
  - chromosome map*

- chromosome theory
- single crossovers*
- **Determining Gene Sequence***
  - multiple crossovers
  - double crossovers*
  - product law*
  - three-point mapping*
  - heterozygous genotype
  - reciprocal classes*
- **Mapping Accuracy***
  - depends on distance*
  - multiple-strand exchanges
  - interference
  - coefficient of coincidence
- **DNA Markers and Computers***
  - useful landmarks

- RFLPs*
- microsatellites*
- short repetitive sequences
- physical map
- **Genetic Exchange**
  - physical exchange
  - chromatids
  - Creighton and McClintock
- sister chromatid exchange*
- mitotic chromosomes
- bromodeoxyuridine
- BrdU
- harlequin chromosomes
- Bloom syndrome
- DNA helicase
- Mendel and Linkage*

F7-1 Illustration of critical arrangements of linked genes. Notice that there are two possible arrangements for an *AaBb* double heterozygote. In order to do linkage problems correctly, such arrangements must be understood.

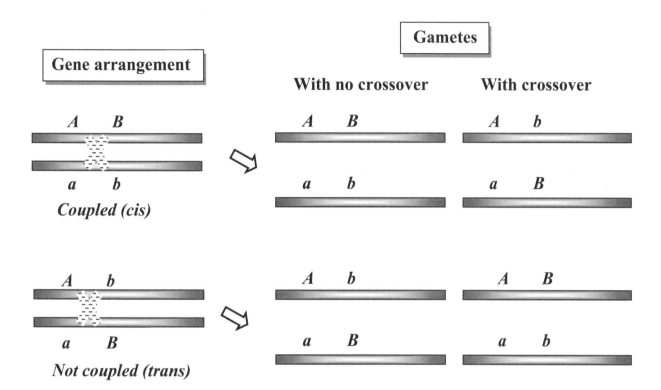

Answers to Now Solve This

7-1. The initial cross for this problem would be

AaBb × *aabb*.

(a) If the two loci are on different chromosomes, independent assortment would occur and the following distribution (1:1:1:1) is expected:

1/4   *AaBb*
1/4   *Aabb*
1/4   *aaBb*
1/4   *aabb*

(b) Even though the two loci are linked and on the same chromosome, the frequency of crossing over is so high that crossovers always occur. Under that condition, independent assortment would occur, and the following distribution (1:1:1:1) is expected:

1/4   *AaBb*
1/4   *Aabb*
1/4   *aaBb*
1/4   *aabb*

(c) If crossovers never occur, then all of the gametes from the heterozygous parent are *parental*. If the arrangement is

AB/ab × *ab/ab*

then the two types of offspring will be as follows:

1/2   *AB/ab*
1/2   *ab/ab*

Under this condition, *AB* are *coupled*. If, however, *A* and *B* are not coupled, then the symbolism would be

Ab/aB × *aabb*

The offspring would occur as follows:

1/2   *Ab/ab*
1/2   *aB/ab*

7-2. Because there is no indication as to the configuration of the *P* and *Z* genes (*coupled or not coupled*) in the parent, one must look at the percentages in the offspring. Notice that the most frequent classes are *PZ* and *pz*. These classes represent the parental (noncrossover) groups, which indicates that the original parental arrangement in the test cross was

PZ/pz × *pz/pz*.

Adding the crossover percentages together (6.9 + 7.1) gives 14 percent, which would be the map distance between the two genes.

7-3. In typical trihybrid crosses, one expects eight kinds of offspring. In this example, only six are listed, and one can assume that because the double crossover class is the least frequent, it is the double crossovers that are not listed.

To work this type of problem, examine the list to see which types are not present. In this case, the double crossover classes are the following:

$+ + c$ and $a\ b\ +$

(a, b) Notice that by comparing the parental classes (most frequent) with the double crossover classes (zero in this case), one can, using the logic of the methods described in the text, determine that the gene b is in the middle and the arrangement is as follows. Note: For consistency, the zeros (double crossovers) are included in the calculations.

$+ b\ c/\ a + +$

$$a - b \quad = \frac{32 + 38 + 0 + 0}{1000} \times 100$$
$$= 7 \text{ map units}$$

$$b - c \quad = \frac{11 + 9 + 0 + 0}{1000} \times 100$$
$$= 2 \text{ map units}$$

(c) The progeny phenotypes that are missing are $+ + c$ and $a\ b\ +$, of which, from 1000 offspring, 1.4 ($0.07 \times 0.02 \times 1000$) would be expected. Perhaps by chance or some other unknown selective factor, they were not observed.

Solutions to Problems and Discussion Questions

1. **(a)** Morgan and his students, especially Alfred Sturtevant, correlated chiasma frequency with the distance between linked genes. The farther apart two genes, the higher the chiasma, and, therefore, crossover frequency. The most important hint was that recombination frequency between genes *a* and *c* could be equal to the recombination frequency between *a* and *b* plus recombination frequency between *b* and *c*.

(b) The discovery of linkage, genes segregating together during gamete formation, indicated a physical association among genes.

(c) Two experimental lines, one using maize (Creighton and McClintock) and the other using *Drosophila*, showed that each time a crossover occurred, an actual physical exchange of chromosomes also occurred. Each experiment demonstrated a switch in chromosomal markers when genetic markers exchanged.

(d) Even when sister chromatid exchanges do not produce new allelic combinations, they can be demonstrated using molecular markers such as bromodeoxyuridine.

2. The biological significance of genetic exchange and recombination appears to be to generate genetic variation in gametes, thereby leading to genetic variation in organisms. By reshuffling genes, new combinations are generated that may then be of evolutionary advantage. In addition, because chromosomal position can influence gene function, variation is created by *position effect*.

3. First, in order for chromosomes to engage in crossing over, they must be in proximity. It is likely that the side-by-side pairing that occurs during synapsis is the earliest time during the cell cycle that chromosomes achieve that necessary proximity. Second, chiasmata are visible during prophase I of meiosis, and it is likely that these structures are intimately associated with the genetic event of crossing over.

4. With some qualification, especially around the centromeres and telomeres, one can say that crossing over is somewhat randomly distributed over the length of the chromosome. Two loci that are far apart are more likely to have a crossover between them than two loci that are close together.

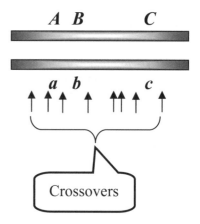

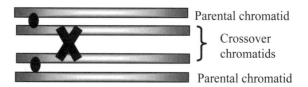

5. Because crossing over occurs at the four-strand stage of the cell cycle (that is, after S phase), notice that each single crossover involves only two (50 percent) of the four chromatids.

6. As mentioned in an earlier answer (4), with some qualifications, crossovers occur randomly along the lengths of chromosomes. Within any region, the occurrence of two events is less likely than the occurrence of one event. If the probability of one event is

$$1/X,$$

the probability of two events occurring at the same time will be

$$1/X^2.$$

7. Positive interference occurs when a crossover in one region of a chromosome interferes with crossovers in nearby regions. Such interference ranges from zero (no interference) to 1.0 (complete interference). Interference is often explained by a physical rigidity of chromatids such that they are unlikely to make sufficiently sharp bends to allow crossovers to be close together.

8. Each cross must be set up in such a way as to reveal crossovers because it is on the basis of crossover frequency that genetic maps are developed. It is necessary that genetic heterogeneity exist so that different arrangements of genes, generated by crossing over, can be distinguished.

The organism that is heterozygous must be the sex in which crossing over occurs. In other words, it would be useless to map genes in *Drosophila* if the male parent is the heterozygote because crossing over is not typical in *Drosophila* males.

Lastly, the cross must be set up so that the phenotypes of the offspring readily reveal their genotypes. The best arrangement is one in which an organism is crossed with another that is fully recessive for the genes being mapped.

9. Because the distance between *dp* and *ap* is greatest, they must be on the "outside" and *cl* must be in the middle. The genetic map would be as follows:

$$dp\text{---}cl\text{--------------------}ap$$

$$3\ mu. \qquad 39\ mu.$$

10. In looking at this problem, one can immediately conclude that the two loci (kernel color and plant color) are linked because the testcross progeny occur in a ratio other than 1:1:1:1 (and epistasis does not appear because all phenotypes expected are present). The question is whether the arrangement in the parents is *coupled*:

$$RY/ry \quad \times \quad ry/ry$$

or *not coupled*:

$$Ry/rY \quad \times \quad ry/ry$$

Notice that the most frequent phenotypes in the offspring, the parentals, are colored, green (88) and colorless, yellow (92). This indicates that the heterozygous parent in the test cross is coupled

$$RY/ry \quad \times \quad ry/ry$$

with the two dominant alleles on one chromosome and the two recessives on the homolog (F7-1). Seeing that there are 20 crossover progeny among the 200, or 20/200, the map distance would be 10 map units (20/200 × 100 to convert to percentages) between the *R* and *Y* loci.

11. Start this problem by working through the expected offspring under two models, one with no crossing over and the second with 30 percent crossing over in the female.

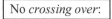

No *crossing over*:

Female gametes:	*Male gametes*:
1/2 *e ca*⁺	1/2 *e ca*⁺
1/2 *e*⁺ *ca*	1/2 *e*⁺ *ca*

Offspring:

1/4	*e* phenotype
2/4	wild
1/4	*ca* phenotype

With 30 percent crossing over:

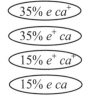 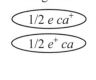

Female gametes:	Male gametes:
35% *e ca*⁺	1/2 *e ca*⁺
35% *e*⁺ *ca*	1/2 *e*⁺ *ca*
15% *e*⁺ *ca*⁺	
15% *e ca*	

Offspring: (obtained by combining gametes and phenotypes)

e phenotype = 17.5% + 7.5%　　**= 25%**

wild phenotype =
17.5% + 7.5% + 17.5% + 7.5% = **50%**

ca phenotype = 17.5% + 7.5%　**= 25%**

Notice that the distribution of phenotypes is the same, regardless of the contribution of the crossover classes.

12. This problem can be approached by looking for the most distant loci (*adp* and *b*) and then filling in the intermediate loci. In this case, the map for parts **(a)** and **(b)** is the following:

d	.........*b*	.........*pr*	.........*vg*	.........*c*	.........*adp*
31	48	54	67	75	83

Map units

The expected map units between *d* and *c* would be 44, between *d* and *vg* 36, and between *d* and *adp* 52. However, because there is a theoretical maximum of 50 map units possible between two loci in any one cross, that distance would be below the 52 determined by simple subtraction.

13.

	female A	*female B*	*Frequency*
NCO	3, 4	7, 8	first
SCO	1, 2	3, 4	second
SCO	7, 8	5, 6	third
DCO	5, 6	1, 2	fourth

The single crossover classes that represent crossovers between the genes that are closer together (d–b) would occur less frequently than the classes of crossovers between more distant genes (b–c).

14. For two reasons, it is clear that the genes are in the *coupled* configuration in the F_1 female. First, a completely homozygous female was mated to a wild-type male, and second, the phenotypes of the offspring indicate the following parental classes

$$sc\ s\ v \text{ and } +++$$

(a)

P_1: $sc\ s\ v / sc\ s\ v \quad \times \quad +++/Y$
F_1: $+++/sc\ s\ v \quad \times \quad sc\ s\ v/Y$

(b) Examine the parental classes (most frequent) and compare the arrangement with the double crossover classes (least frequent). Notice that the v gene "switches places" between the two groups (parentals and double crossovers). The gene that switches places is in the middle.

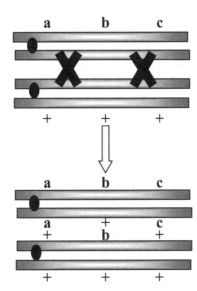

The map distances are determined by first writing the proper arrangement and sequence of genes, and then computing the distances between each set of genes.

$$\frac{sc\ v\ s}{+++}$$

$$sc - v = \frac{150 + 156 + 10 + 14}{1000} \times 100$$

$$= 33 \text{ percent (map units)}$$

$$v - s = \frac{46 + 30 + 10 + 14}{1000} \times 100$$

$$= 10 \text{ percent (map units)}$$

Double crossovers are always added into each crossover group because they represent a crossover in each region.

$$\underbrace{sc\text{-------}}_{33}\underbrace{v\text{-----}s}_{10}$$

(c, d) The coefficient of coincidence =

$$\frac{\text{observed freq. double C/O}}{\text{expected freq. double C/O}}$$

$$= \frac{(14 + 10)/1000}{0.33 \times 0.1}$$

$$= \frac{0.024}{0.033} = 0.727$$

which indicates that there were fewer double crossovers than expected; therefore, positive chromosomal interference is present.

15. This setup involves an F_1 in which the fully heterozygous female has the genes y and w in *coupled* and *ct not coupled*. The arrangement for the cross is, therefore,

(a) $y\ w\ +/+ + ct \quad \times \quad y\ w\ +/Y$

It is important at this point to determine the gene sequence. Using methods I or II, examine the parental classes and compare the arrangement with the double crossover (least frequent) classes. Notice that the w gene "switches places" between the two groups (parentals and double crossovers). The gene that switches places is in the middle. Therefore, the arrangement as written above is correct.

(b)

$$y - w = \frac{9 + 6 + 0 + 0}{1000} \times 100$$

$$= 1.5 \text{ map units}$$

$$w - ct = \frac{90 + 95 + 0 + 0}{1000} \times 100$$

$$= 18.5 \text{ map units}$$

```
y-------------- w----------------------------ct
0.0              1.5                          20.0
```

(c) There were

$$0.185 \times 0.015 \times 1000 = 2.775$$

double crossovers expected.

(d) Because the cross to the F_1 males included the normal (wild-type) allele for *cut wings*, it would not be possible to unequivocally determine the genotypes from the F_2 phenotypes for all classes.

16. (a) The cross will be as follows. Represent the *Dichaete* gene as an uppercase letter because it is dominant.

P_1:	$D + +/+ + +$	$\times$	$+ e\ p/+ e\ p$	
F_1:	$D + +/+ e\ p$	$\times$	$+ e\ p/+ e\ p$	
F_2:	$D + +/+ e\ p$	Dichaete		
	$+ e\ p /+ e\ p$	ebony, pink		
	$D e +/+ e\ p$	Dichaete, ebony		
	$+ + p/+ e\ p$	pink		
	$D + p/+ e\ p$	Dichaete, pink		
	$+ e +/+ e\ p$	ebony		
	$D e\ p/+ e\ p$	Dichaete, ebony, pink		
	$+ + +/+ e\ p$	wild-type		

(b) Determine which gene is in the middle by comparing the parental classes with the double crossover classes. Notice that the *pink* gene "switches places" between the two groups (parentals and double crossovers). The gene that switches places is in the middle. So rewriting the sequence of genes with the correct arrangement gives the following:

F_1:	$D + +/+ p\ e$ $\times$ $+ p\ e/+ p\ e$

Distances: remember to add in the double crossover classes

$$D - p = \frac{12 + 13 + 2 + 3}{1000} \times 100$$

$$= 3.0 \text{ map units}$$

$$p - e = \frac{84 + 96 + 2 + 3}{1000} \times 100$$

$$= 18.5 \text{ map units}$$

17. Because two of the genes are linked and 20 map units apart on the third chromosome, and one is on the second chromosome, the problem is a combination of linkage and independent assortment. First provide the genotypes of the parents in the original cross and the reciprocal. Use a semicolon to indicate that two different chromosome pairs are involved.

P_1:
females: $+/+$; $p\ e/p\ e$
$\times$
males: dp/dp; $+ +/+ +$

F_1:
females: $+/dp$; $+ +/p\ e$
$\times$
males: dp/dp; $p\ e/p\ e$

Female gametes: Use a modification of the forked-line method for determining the types of gametes to be produced. The *dumpy* locus will give $0.5 +$ and $0.5\ dp$ to the gametes because of independent assortment (on a different chromosome), and the other two loci will segregate with 20 percent (map units) being the recombinants and 80 percent being the parentals.

	$0.4 +$	$+$ (parental)	$= 0.20 + + +$
$0.5 +$	$0.1 +$	e (crossover)	$= 0.05 + + e$
	$0.1\ p$	$+$ (crossover)	$= 0.05 + p +$
	$0.4\ p$	e (parental)	$= 0.20 + p\ e$

	$0.4 +$	$+$ (parental)	$= 0.20\ dp + +$
	$0.1 +$	e (crossover)	$= 0.05\ dp + e$
$0.5\ dp$	$0.1\ p$	$+$ (crossover)	$= 0.05\ dp\ p +$
	$0.4\ p$	e (parental)	$= 0.20\ dp\ p\ e$

Crossed with $dp\ p\ e$ from the male gives the following offspring:

0.20 wild-type
0.05 ebony
0.05 pink
0.20 pink, ebony
0.20 dumpy
0.05 dumpy, ebony
0.05 dumpy, pink
0.20 dumpy, pink, ebony

For the reciprocal cross:

F$_1$:

males: $+/dp$; $++/p$ e

×

females: dp/dp; p e/p e

there would be no crossover classes.

0.5 + ⟋ 0.5 +   + (parental) = 0.25 + + +
0.5 + — 0.5 p e (parental) = 0.25 + p e

0.5 dp ⟋ 0.5 +   + (parental) = 0.25 dp + +
0.5 dp — 0.5 p e (parental) = 0.25 dp p e

Crossing with dp p e from the female gives the following offspring:

0.25 wild-type
0.25 pink, ebony
0.25 dumpy
0.25 dumpy, pink, ebony

The results would change because of the absence of crossing over in males.

18. Because *Stubble* is a dominant mutation (and homozygous lethal), one can determine whether it is heterozygous (*Sb*/+) or homozygous wild-type (+/+). One would use the typical testcross arrangement with the *curled* gene so the male parent arrangement would be

$+$ $cu/+$ cu

19. First make a drawing with the genes placed on the homologous chromosomes as follows:

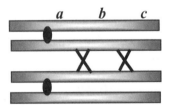

Realize that there are four chromatids in each tetrad and a single crossover involves only two of the four chromatids. Noninvolved chromatids must be added to the non-crossover classes. Do all the crossover classes first, then add up the non-crossover chromatids. For example, in the first crossover class (20 between *a* and *b*), notice that there will be 40 chromatids that were not involved in the crossover. These 40 must be added to the *abc* and +++ classes.

$a\,b\,c$ = 168
$+++$ = 168
$a++$ = 20
$+\,b\,c$ = 20
$++\,c$ = 10
$a\,b+$ = 10
$+\,b+$ = 2
$a+c$ = 2

The map distances would be computed as follows:

$$a-b = \frac{20+20+2+2}{400}\times100$$
$$= 11 \text{ map units}$$

$$b-c = \frac{10+10+2+2}{400}\times100$$
$$= 6 \text{ map units}$$

20. Assign the following symbols, for example:

R = Red r = yellow
O = Oval o = long

Progeny A: $Ro/rO \times rroo$ = 10 map units
Progeny B: $RO/ro \times rroo$ = 10 map units

21. (a) There are several ways to think through this problem. Remember that there is no crossing over in *Drosophila* males. Therefore, any gene on the same chromosome will be completely linked to any other gene on the same chromosome. Because you can get *pink* by itself, *short* cannot be completely linked to it. This leaves linkage to *black* on the second chromosome, the fourth chromosome, or the X chromosome. Because the distribution of phenotypes in males and females is essentially the same, the gene cannot be X-linked. In addition, the F$_1$ males were wild, and if the *short* gene is on the X, the F$_1$ males would be short.

It is also reasonable to state that the gene cannot be on the fourth chromosome because there would be eight phenotypic classes (independent assortment of three genes) instead of the four observed. Through these insights, one could conclude that the *short* gene is on chromosome 2 with the *black* gene.

Another way to approach this problem is to make three chromosomal configurations possible in the F$_1$ male. By producing gametes from this male, the answer becomes obvious.

Case A	Case B	Case C
p b *sh*	*p sh* *b*	*b sh* *p*
+ + +	+ + +	+ + +

Develop the gametes from case C and cross them out to the completely recessive triple mutant. You will get the results in the table.

(b) The parental cross is now the following:

> Females: *b sh p* × Males: *b sh p*
>   + +   +   *b sh p*

The new gametes resulting from crossing over in the female would be *b* + and + *sh*. Because the gene *p* is assorting independently, it is not important in this discussion. Because 15 percent of the offspring now contain these recombinant chromatids, the map distance between the two genes must be 15.

22. Notice that in the description of the genotype of the female, no mention is made of the *cis-trans* (coupling-repulsion) arrangement of the genes. The data will supply that information. Begin with a set of symbols as indicated below:

B^+ = wild eye shape
B = Bar eye shape

m^+ = wild wings
m = miniature wings

e^+ = wild body color
e = ebony body color

Superficially, the cross would be as follows:

$B^+B \ m^+m \ e^+e \ \times \ B^+? \ m? \ e?$

(The *?* is used at this point to indicate that we have no information allowing us to decide whether any of the alleles in the male are X-linked.)

Notice from the data that there are approximately as many ebony offspring (282) as those with wild body color (283). Therefore, we can conclude that the *ebony* locus is not linked to *B* or *m*. Notice also that the most frequent offspring regarding eye shape and wing size are wild-miniature and Bar-wild. This suggests that the arrangement is "trans" or "repulsion," as indicated below:

$B \ m^+/B^+m; \ e^+/e$

Notice that a semicolon is used to indicate that the *ebony* locus is on a different chromosome. At this point and without prior knowledge, we still don't know whether any of the genes are X-linked; however, it is of no consequence to the solution of the problem. (In actuality, both *B* and *m* loci are X-linked.) To determine the map distances (again, *ebony* is out

of the mapping picture at this point because it is not linked to either *B* or *m*):

111 + 115 = 226	= parental
117 + 101 = 218	= parental
26 + 31 = 57	= crossover
29 + 35 = 64	= crossover

Mapping the distance between *B* and *m* would be as follows:

$$(57 + 64)/ (226 + 218 + 57 + 64) \times 100 =$$
$$121/565 \times 100 \ = 21.4 \text{ map units.}$$

We would conclude that the *ebony* locus is either far away from *B* and *m* (50 map units or more) or it is on a different chromosome. In fact, *ebony* is on a different chromosome.

23. (a) There would be $2^n = 8$ genotypic and phenotypic classes, and they would occur in a 1:1:1:1:1:1:1:1 ratio.

(b) There would be two classes, and they would occur in a 1:1 ratio.

(c) There are 20 map units between the *A* and *B* loci, and locus *C* assorts independently from both the *A* and *B* loci.

24. Because the genetic map is more accurate when relatively small distances are covered and when large numbers of offspring are scored, this map would probably not be too accurate with such a small sample size.

25. The purpose of the experiment was to determine whether genetic crossing over involved actual physical exchange of chromosomal material. Other models of the time did not necessarily require an actual physical rearrangement of chromosomal material during recombination. By having microscopically visible markers on the chromosomes, Creighton and McClintock were able to show that homologous chromosomal material physically exchanged segments during crossing over.

26. In contrast to the other organisms mentioned, a single human mating pair produces relatively few offspring and the haploid number of chromosomes is relatively high (23), so there are rather small numbers of identifiable genes per chromosome. In addition, accurate medical records are often difficult to obtain and the life cycle is relatively long.

27. DNA markers are unique DNA sequences whose sequence and chromosomal location are known. They serve as landmarks for the mapping of genes. Typical markers include restriction fragment length polymorphisms (RFLPs), microsatellites, and single nucleotide polymorphisms (SNPs). Because the number of DNA markers in an individual may be in the tens of thousands, they can "mark" small intervals of each of the 23 human chromosomes.

28. Because sister chromatids are genetically identical (with the exception of rare new mutations), crossing over between sisters provides no increase in genetic variability.

Chapter 8: Genetic Analysis and Mapping in Bacteria and Bacteriophages

Concept Areas	Corresponding Problems
Genetic Recombination in Bacteria	1, 2, 3
Conjugation	1, 2, 3, 4, 5, 6, 7, 8, 16
Transformation	2, 9
Bacteriophages	10, 11, 12, 13, 14, 15, 20, 21, 22
Transduction	1, 2, 17, 18, 19
Mutation and Recombination in Viruses	1

Structures and Processes Checklist – Significant concepts that deserve special attention are identified with a "*".

(check topic when mastered – provide examples where appropriate – understand the context of each entry)

- **Bacteria and Bacteriophages**
  - recombination*
- **Bacteria Mutate**
  - minimal medium*
  - prototroph*
  - auxotroph*
  - serial dilution*
  - dilution factor*
- **Genetic Recombination***
  - conjugation*
  - F$^+$ cells*
  - F$^-$ cells*
  - F pilus
  - sex pilus
  - fertility factor*
  - Hfr bacteria*
  - chromosome mapping

- *E. coli* K12
- high-frequency recombination*
- interrupted mating*
- oriented transfer*
- map based on time*
- origin of transfer*
- F' state*
- merozygote
- **Rec Proteins Are Essential***
  - RecA protein
  - single-stranded displacement
- **F Factor and Plasmids***
  - R plasmids*
  - resistance transfer factor
  - RTF
  - Col plasmid
  - ColE1

Chapter 8 Genetic Analysis and Mapping in Bacteria and Bacteriophages

- ○ colicins
- ○ **Transformation***
  - ○ competence
  - ○ donor DNA
  - ○ homologous region*
  - ○ heteroduplex
  - ○ transformation and linkage*
- ○ **Bacteriophages***
  - ○ phages
  - ○ phage T4
  - ○ plaque assay*
  - ○ plaque
  - ○ lysogeny*
  - ○ prophage*
  - ○ temperate phages*
- ○ virulent phages*
- ○ lysogenic*
- ○ episome
- ○ **Transduction***
  - ○ virus-mediated transfer
  - ○ *Salmonella typhimurium*
  - ○ auxotrophic strains*
  - ○ P22
  - ○ lysis
  - ○ nature of transduction*
  - ○ mapping*
  - ○ cotransduction*
- ○ **Intergenic Recombination***
  - ○ bacteriophage mutations
  - ○ mixed infection experiments*

Answers to Now Solve This

8-1. One can approach this problem by lining up the data from the various crosses in the following order:

Hfr Strain	*Order*
1	*t c h r o*
2	*h r o m b*
3	*<<c h r o m*
4	*m b a k t>>*
5	*<<b a k t c*

Overall: | *t c h r o m b a k*

Notice that all of the genes can be linked to give a consistent map and that the ends overlap, indicating that the map is circular. The order is reversed in two of the crosses, indicating the orientation of transfer is reversed.

8-2. In the first data set, the transformation of each locus, a^+ and b^+, occurs at a frequency of 0.031 and 0.012, respectively. To determine whether there is linkage, one would determine whether the frequency of double transformants a^+b^+ is greater than that expected by a multiplication of the two independent events. Multiplying 0.031×0.012 gives 0.00037, or approximately 0.04 percent. From this information, one would consider no linkage between these two loci. Notice that this frequency is approximately the same as the frequency in the second experiment, in which the loci are transformed independently.

Chapter 8 Genetic Analysis and Mapping in Bacteria and Bacteriophages

Solutions to Problems and Discussion Questions

1. (a) A variety of experiments involving transformation, conjugation, and transduction showed that genetic elements from one bacterial strain can be transferred to another strain. Historically, transformation set the stage for the discovery that DNA is the genetic material in bacteria.

(b) The general strategy for determining the dependence of cell-to-cell contact in one form of bacterial recombination involved a Davis U-tube and a filter. When the filter separated two auxotrophic strains, no genetic recombination occurred.

(c) A filterable agent was discovered such that when two auxotrophic strains were placed on opposite sides of a Davis U-tube apparatus, there was a one-way passage of genetic material. The filterable agent was insensitive to DNase treatment and was therefore not naked DNA. Bacterial contact was eliminated by the filter.

(d) Intergenic recombination in bacteriophages was demonstrated by mixed infections that yielded recombinants. Such recombinants can be used in mapping of genes.

2. Three modes of recombination in bacteria are *conjugation*, *transformation*, and *transduction*. Conjugation is dependent on the F factor, which, by a variety of mechanisms, can direct genetic exchange between two bacterial cells. Transformation is the uptake of exogenous DNA by cells. Transduction is the exchange of genetic material using a bacteriophage.

3. (a) The requirement for physical contact between bacterial cells during conjugation was established by placing a filter in a U-tube such that the medium can be exchanged but the bacteria cannot come in contact. Under this condition, conjugation does not occur.

(b) By treating cells with streptomycin, an antibiotic, it was shown that recombination would not occur if one of the two bacterial strains was inactivated. However, if the other was similarly treated, recombination would occur. Thus, directionality was suggested, with one strain being a donor strain and the other being the recipient.

(c) An F^+ bacterium contains a circular, double-stranded, structurally independent DNA molecule, the F^+ factor plasmid, that can direct recombination.

4. In an $F^+ \times F^-$ cross, the transfer of the F factor produces a recipient bacterium that is F^+. Any gene may be transferred, and the frequency of transfer is relatively low. Crosses that are $Hfr \times F^-$ produce recombinants at a higher frequency than the $F^+ \times F^-$ cross. The transfer is oriented (nonrandom) and the recipient cell remains F^-.

5. Bacteria that are F^+ possess the F factor, while those that are F^- lack the F factor. In Hfr cells, the F factor is integrated into the bacterial chromosome; in F' bacteria, the F factor is free of the bacterial chromosome yet possesses a piece of the bacterial chromosome.

6. Mapping the chromosome in an $Hfr \times F^-$ cross takes advantage of the oriented transfer of the bacterial chromosome through the conjugation tube. For each F type, the point of insertion and the direction of transfer are fixed; therefore, breaking the conjugation tube at different times produces partial diploids with corresponding portions of the donor chromosome being transferred. The length of the chromosome being transferred is contingent on the duration of conjugation, thus mapping of genes is based on time.

7. In an $Hfr \times F^-$ cross, the F factor is directing the transfer of the donor chromosome. It takes approximately 90 minutes to transfer the entire chromosome. Because the F factor is the last element to be transferred and the conjugation tube is fragile, the likelihood for complete transfer is low.

8. As shown in the text, the F^+ element can enter the host bacterial chromosome, and upon returning to its independent state, it may pick up a piece of a bacterial chromosome. When transferred to a bacterium with a complete chromosome, a partial diploid, or merozygote, is formed.

9. Transformation requires *competence* on the part of the recipient bacterium, meaning that only under certain conditions are bacterial cells capable of being transformed. Transforming DNA must initially be *double-stranded* to begin with, yet it is converted to a single-stranded structure upon insertion into the host cell. The most efficient length of the transforming DNA is about 1/200 of the size of the host chromosome. Transformation is an energy-requiring process, and the number of sites on the bacterial cell surface is limited.

10. The phage not only lacks genes for ribosomal construction, but also contains no ribosomes. Upon infection, phage genes are transcribed and the transcripts are translated using bacterial ribosomes.

11. Depending on the particular phage, the life cycle is generally initiated when the virus binds by adsorption to the bacterial host cell. Contraction of the tail sheath causes the central core to cross the cell wall. The DNA in the head is injected through the cell membrane into the bacterium. Bacterial DNA, RNA, and protein synthesis are inhibited, and synthesis of viral RNAs begins using bacterial machinery. Degradation of the host DNA is initiated. Phage DNA replication occurs, leading to a pool of viral DNA molecules. The components of the head, tail, and tail fibers are then synthesized. Three sequential pathways occur to assemble the progeny phage:

(1) DNA packaging as the viral heads are assembled,

(2) tail assembly, and

(3) tail fiber assembly.

After DNA is packaged into the head, it combines with the tail components, and the tail fibers are added.

12. A single plaque originates from the replicative activity of a single bacteriophage.

13. A single plaque is a clearing of bacteria resulting from the lytic action of millions of bacteriophage.

14. Notice that each of the serial dilutions is hundred-fold, and three dilutions were made. This leads to a final $10^{-2} \times 10^{-2} \times 10^{-2} = 10^{-6}$ dilution. Assuming the typical introduction of 0.1 ml of the phage suspension to the bacterial solution, because 17 plaques were formed, the initial density of bacteriophage suspension would be calculated as follows:

170 phage/ml $\times 10^6 = 1.7 \times 10^8$ phage/ml

15. A lytic cycle occurs as bacteriophages enter a bacterial host and form progeny phages after a relatively short period of time. There is no extensive latent period, in that progeny may be produced within an hour or two. *Lysogeny* is a complex process whereby certain temperate phage can enter a bacterial cell and, instead of following a lytic developmental path, integrate their DNA into the bacterial chromosome. In doing so, the bacterial cell becomes lysogenic. The latent, integrated phage chromosome is called a *prophage*.

16. A prophage is the latent, noninfective state of the bacteriophage chromosome when it is incorporated into the host bacterial chromosome.

17. In their experiment, a filter was placed between the two auxotrophic strains, which would not allow contact. F-mediated conjugation requires contact, and without that contact, such conjugation cannot occur. The treatment with DNase showed that the filterable agent was not naked DNA.

18. In *generalized transduction,* virtually any genetic element from a host strain may be included in the phage coat and thereby be transduced. In *specialized transduction*, only certain genes are transduced.

19. The first problem to be solved is the gene order. Clearly, the parental types are

$$a^+b^+c^+ \text{ and } a^-b^-c^-$$

because they are the most frequent. The least frequent are the double crossover types:

$$a^-b^-c^+ \text{ and } a^+b^+c^-.$$

Because it is the gene in the middle that switches places when one compares the parental and double crossover classes, the c gene must be in the middle.

The map distances are as follows:

a to c $\quad = (740 + 670 + 90 + 110)/10,000$

$\quad\quad\quad = 16.1$ map units

c to b $\quad = (160 + 140 + 90 + 110)/10,000$

$\quad\quad\quad = 5$ map units

20. Viral recombination occurs when there is a sufficiently high number of infecting viruses so that there is a high likelihood that more than one variant of phage will infect a given bacterium. Under this condition, phage chromosomes can recombine by crossing over.

21. Starting with a single bacteriophage, one lytic cycle produces 200 progeny phages; three more lytic cycles would produce $(200)^4$ or 1,600,000,000 phages.

22. (a) Remembering that 0.1 ml is typically used in the plaque assay, the initial concentration of phage per milliliter is greater than 10^5.

(b) Remembering that 0.1 ml is typically used in the plaque assay, the initial concentration of phage per milliliter is around 140×10^5 or 1.4×10^7.

(c) Remembering that 0.1 ml is typically used in the plaque assay, the initial concentration of phage is less than 10^7. Coupling this information with the calculations in part (b) above, it would appear that the initial concentration of phage is around 1×10^7, and the failure to obtain plaques in this portion of the experiment is expected and due to sampling error.

Chapter 9: DNA Structure and Analysis

Concept Areas	Corresponding Problems
Central Dogma	1, 2, 8
Transformation	3, 4, 5
Differential Labeling	6, 7
Genetic Variation	2, 28, 29
Model Building	1, 10, 14, 15, 16, 17, 27, 30
Nucleic Acid Structure	1, 10, 11, 12, 13, 14, 26
Analytical Methods	7, 20, 21, 22, 23, 24, 31, 32, 33
Replication	2, 25
RNA as Genetic Material	9, 18, 19

Structures and Processes Checklist – Significant concepts that deserve special attention are identified with a "*".

(check topic when mastered – provide examples where appropriate – understand the context of each entry)

- **Genetic Material**
  - Watson and Crick*
- **Four Characteristics***
  - replication*
  - storage of information*
  - expression of information*
  - variation by mutation*
  - transcription*
  - mRNA
  - rRNA
  - tRNA
  - central dogma*
- **1944***
  - nuclein
  - tetranucleotide hypothesis

- **Evidence Favoring DNA***
  - transformation studies*
  - virulent strains
  - avirulent strains
  - smooth colonies
  - rough colonies
  - serotypes
  - *Diplococcus*
  - II*R*
  - III*S*
  - transformation*
  - transforming principle*
  - *in vitro*
  - *in vivo*
  - highly purified DNA*

- ribonuclease*
- protease*
- deoxyribonuclease*
- Hershey-Chase experiment*
- bacteriophage
- T2
- phage
- 50 percent protein*
- 50 percent DNA*
- ^{32}P*
- ^{35}S*
- blender*
- phage "ghosts"
- transfection experiments*
- protoplasts
- spheroplasts
- transfection

- **Indirect and Direct Evidence***
  - *n, 2n**
  - mutation action spectrum*
  - absorption spectrum*
  - mutagenic wavelengths*
  - recombinant DNA studies*
  - recombinant DNA technology
  - transgenic animals
  - *β*-globin gene

- **RNA as Genetic Material***
  - tobacco mosaic virus*
  - TMV

- retrovirus*
- reverse transcription*
- reverse transcriptase
- HIV

- **Structure of DNA***
  - base composition*
  - X-ray diffraction studies*
  - model building*
  - *The Double Helix**
  - nitrogenous base*
  - pentose sugar*
  - phosphate group*
  - purine*
  - pyramidine*
  - adenine*
  - guanine*
  - cytosine*
  - thymine*
  - uracil*
  - ribonucleic acids (RNA)*
  - deoxyribonucleic acids (DNA)*
  - ribose*
  - deoxyribose*
  - C-2' position*
  - 2-deoxyribose
  - nucleoside
  - nucleotide
  - nucleoside monophosphate
  - NMP

- nucleoside diphosphate
- NDP
- adenosine triphosphate*
- ATP
- guanosine triphosphate*
- GTP
- inorganic phosphate
- P_i
- phosphodiester bond*
- oligonucleotide
- polynucleotide
- base composition*
- proportionality*
- $(A + G) = (C + T)$*
- $(G + C)/(A + T)$ varies*
- X-ray diffraction*
- Watson-Crick model*
- right-handed double helix
- bases stacked
- 0.34 nm
- $A = T, G = C$
- minor groove
- major groove
- 2.0 nm
- bases paired
- complementarity*
- hydrogen bond*
- hydrophobic*
- hydrophilic*
- semiconservative replication*

- **Alternative DNA Forms**
  - A-DNA
  - B-DNA
  - single-crystal analysis
  - Z-DNA
  - left-handed helix
  - RNA structure*
  - ribosomal RNA*
  - rRNA
  - messenger RNA*
  - mRNA
  - transfer RNA*
  - tRNA
  - Svedberg coefficient
  - ribosomes
  - telomerase RNA
  - small nuclear RNA
  - snRNA
  - antisense RNA
  - microRNA
  - miRNA
  - short interfering RNA
  - siRNA
- **Analytical Techniques***
  - hyperchromic shift*
  - melting temperature*
  - T_m
  - molecular hybridization*
  - denaturation

85

Chapter 9 DNA Structure and Analysis

- renaturation
- GC base pairs*
- three hydrogen bonds*
- probe*
- in situ hybridization*
- FISH*
- reassociation kinetics*

- repetitive sequences*
- heating and denaturation*
- unique DNA sequences*
- electrophoresis*
- polyacrylamide gel*
- agarose gel*
- blotting*

F9-1 Illustration of relationships between DNA, its functions, and related products.

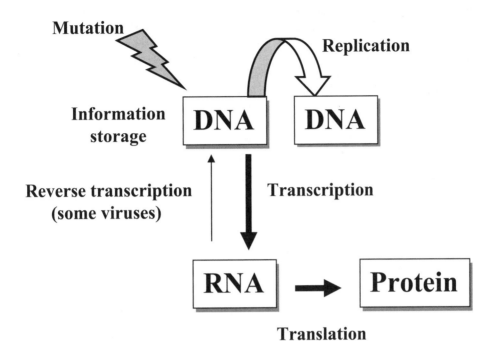

Answers to Now Solve This

9-1. In theory, the general design would be appropriate in that some substance, if labeled, would show up in the progeny of transformed bacteria. However, because the amount of transforming DNA is extremely small compared to the genomic DNA of the recipient bacterium and its progeny, it would be technically difficult to assay for the labeled nucleic acid. In addition, it would be necessary to know that the small stretch of DNA that caused the genetic transformation was actually labeled. This in itself would be relatively easy using present-day recombinant DNA techniques; however, in earlier times, such specific labeling would have been difficult.

9-2. Guanine = 17.5 percent, adenine and thymine both = 32.5 percent.

9-3. Assuming the value of 1.13 is statistically different from 1.00, one can conclude that rubella is a single-stranded RNA virus.

Chapter 9 DNA Structure and Analysis

Solutions to Problems and Discussion Questions

1. (a) Major lines of evidence that DNA is the genetic material originally came from experiments using bacteria and bacteriophages. Transformation studies showed that DNA is the genetic material in bacteria and differential labeling (proteins and nucleic acids) of bacteriophage T2 showed that DNA is the genetic material in some viruses. Both direct and indirect studies have shown that DNA is the genetic material in eukaryotes. Other than in mitochondria and chloroplasts, DNA is localized in the nucleus, where its quantity varies with ploidy (*n*, 2*n*) as one would predict for the genetic material. In addition, the action spectrum of UV light overlaps the absorption spectrum of DNA. Direct evidence comes from recombinant DNA studies in which transgenic organisms can be generated with transferred DNA.

(b) A right-handed double helix with antiparallel polynucleotide chains was first proposed by Watson and Crick. The constant diameter of the DNA double helix and its greatest stability in a right-handed form add additional support.

(c) Given base composition studies showing proportional amounts of A and T, and G and C, and X-ray diffraction studies, Watson and Crick showed that hydrogen bonding configurations between the bases provided attraction and stability for a DNA double helix.

(d) Rapidly renaturing sequences were discovered by Britten and Kohne. They suggested and later showed that such sequences were repetitive.

2. *Replication* is the process that leads to the production of identical copies of the existing genetic information. Because daughter cells contain essentially exact copies (with some exceptions) of genetic information of the parent cell, and through the production and union of gametes, offspring contain copies (with variation) of parental genetic information, the genetic material must copy (replicate) itself. Replication is accomplished during the S phase of interphase in eukaryotes.

The genetic material is capable of *expression* through the production of a phenotype. Through transcription and translation, proteins are produced that contribute to the phenotype of the organism. The genetic material must be stable enough to maintain information in *storage* from one cell to the next and one organism to the next. Because the genetic

material is not "used up" in the processes of transcription and translation, genetic information can be stored and used constantly.

Above, it was stated that the genetic material must be stable enough to store genetic information; however, variation through *mutation* provides the raw material for evolution. The genetic material is capable of a variety of changes, both at the chromosomal and nucleotide levels. See F9-1.

3. Prior to 1940, most of the interest in genetics centered on the transmission of similarity and variation from parents to offspring (transmission genetics). Whereas some experiments examined the possible nature of the hereditary material, abundant knowledge of the structural and enzymatic properties of proteins generated a bias that worked to favor proteins as the hereditary substance.

In addition, proteins were composed of as many as 20 different subunits (amino acids), thereby providing ample structural and functional variation for the multiple tasks that must be accomplished by the genetic material. The tetranucleotide hypothesis (about DNA structure) provided insufficient variability to account for the diverse roles of the genetic material.

4. Griffith performed experiments with different strains of *Diplococcus pneumoniae* in which a heat-killed pathogen, when injected into a mouse with a live nonpathogenic strain, eventually led to the mouse's death. A summary of this experiment is provided in the text. Examination of the dead mouse revealed living pathogenic bacteria. Griffith suggested that the heat-killed virulent (pathogenic) bacteria transformed the avirulent (nonpathogenic) strain into a virulent strain. Alloway showed that a chemical extract of the virulent cells was sufficient to cause transformation of avirulent cells, further reinforcing the hypothesis that the transforming factor has a chemical basis. Avery and coworkers systematically searched for the transforming principle originating from the heat-killed pathogenic strain and determined it to be DNA. Others showed that transformed bacteria are capable of serving as donors of transforming DNA, indicating that the process of transformation involves a stable alteration in the genetic material (DNA).

5. Transformation is dependent on a macromolecule (DNA) that can be extracted and purified from bacteria. During such purification, however, other macromolecular species may contaminate the DNA. Specific degradative enzymes, proteases, RNase, and DNase were used to selectively eliminate components of the extract and, if transformation is concomitantly eliminated, then the eliminated fraction is the transforming principle. DNase eliminates DNA and transformation; therefore, it must be the transforming principle.

6. Nucleic acids contain large amounts of phosphorus and no sulfur, whereas proteins contain sulfur and no phosphorus. Therefore, the radioisotopes ^{32}P and ^{35}S will selectively label nucleic acids and proteins, respectively.

The Hershey and Chase experiment is based on the premise that the substance injected into the bacterium is the substance responsible for producing the progeny phages and therefore must be the hereditary material. The experiment demonstrated that most of the ^{32}P-labeled material (DNA) was injected whereas the phage ghosts (protein coats) remained outside the bacterium. Therefore, the nucleic acid must be the genetic material.

7. Actually, phosphorus is found in approximately equal amounts in DNA and RNA. Therefore, labeling with ^{32}P would "tag" both RNA and DNA. However, the T2 phage, in its mature state, contains very little if any RNA; therefore, DNA would be interpreted as being the genetic material in T2 phage.

8. The early evidence would be considered indirect in that at no time was there an experiment, like transformation in bacteria, in which genetic information in one organism was transferred to another using DNA. Rather, by comparing DNA content in various cell types (sperm and somatic cells) and observing that the *action* and *absorption* spectra of ultraviolet light were correlated, DNA was considered to be the genetic material. This suggestion was supported by the fact that DNA was shown to be the genetic material in bacteria and some phage. Direct evidence for DNA being the genetic material comes from a variety of observations, including gene transfer that has been facilitated by recombinant DNA techniques.

9. Some viruses contain a genetic material composed of RNA. The tobacco mosaic virus is composed of an RNA core and a protein coat. "Crosses" can be made in which the protein coat and RNA of TMV are interchanged with another strain (Holmes ribgrass).

The source of the RNA determines the type of lesion; thus, RNA is the genetic material in these viruses. Retroviruses contain RNA as the genetic material and use an enzyme known as *reverse transcriptase* to produce DNA, which can be integrated into the host chromosome. See F9-1. Note: The term "organism" generally refers to membrane-bound, nonviral, living systems. Therefore, technically all organisms have DNA as their genetic material.

10. The structure of deoxyadenylic acid is given below and in the text. Linkages among the three components require the removal of water (H_2O).

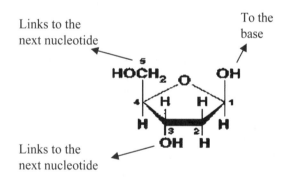

11. The numbering of the carbons on the sugar is especially important (see diagram below). Examine the text for the numbers on the carbons and nitrogens of the bases:

Links to the next nucleotide

To the base

Links to the next nucleotide

12. Examine the structures of the bases in the text. The other bases would be named as follows:

Guanine:	2-amino-6-oxypurine
Cytosine:	2-oxy-4-aminopyrimidine
Thymine:	2, 4-dioxy-5-methylpyrimidine
Uracil:	2, 4-dioxypyrimidine

13. Examine the text for the format for this drawing. Note that the complementary strand must be drawn in the antiparallel orientation.

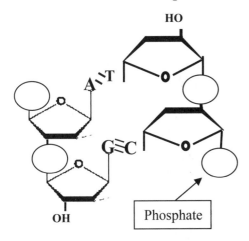

14. The following are characteristics of the Watson-Crick double-helix model for DNA:

The base composition is such that A = T, G = C and (A + G) = (C + T). Bases are stacked, 0.34 nm (3.4 Angstroms) apart, in a plectonic, antiparallel manner. There is one complete turn for each 3.4 nm, which constitutes 10 bases per turn. Hydrogen bonds hold the two polynucleotide chains together, each being formed by phosphodiester linkages between the five-carbon sugars and the phosphates. There are two hydrogen bonds forming the A to T pair and three forming the G to C pair. The double helix exists as a twisted structure, approximately 20 Angstroms in diameter, with a topography of major and minor grooves. The hydrophobic bases are located in the center of the molecule, whereas the hydrophilic phosphodiester backbone is on the outside.

15. In addition to creative "genius" and perseverance, model-building skills, and the conviction that the structure would turn out to be "simple" and have a natural beauty in its simplicity, Watson and Crick employed the X-ray diffraction information of Franklin and Wilkins, the base ratio information of Chargaff, and the knowledge of the nucleotide structures.

16. Because in double-stranded DNA, A = T and G = C (within limits of experimental error), the data presented would have indicated a lack of pairing of these bases in favor of a single-stranded structure or some other nonhydrogen-bonded structure.

Alternatively, from the data, it would appear that A = C and T = G, which would negate the chance for typical hydrogen bonding because opposite charge

relationships do not exist. Therefore, it is quite unlikely that a tight helical structure would form at all.

17. A covalent bond is a relatively strong bond that involves the sharing of electrons between two or more atoms. Hydrogen bonds, much weaker than covalent bonds, are formed as a result of

electrostatic attraction between a covalently bonded hydrogen atom and an atom with an unshared electron pair. The hydrogen atom assumes a partial positive charge, while the unshared electron pair—characteristic of covalently bonded oxygen and nitrogen atoms— assumes a partial negative charge. These opposite charges are responsible for the weak chemical attraction. (Klug et al.)

Complementarity, responsible for the chemical attraction between adenine and thymine (uracil in RNA) and guanine and cytosine, is responsible for DNA and RNA assuming its double-stranded character. Complementarity is based on hydrogen bonding.

18. Three main differences between RNA and DNA are the following:

(1) uracil in RNA replaces thymine in DNA,
(2) ribose in RNA replaces deoxyribose in DNA, and
(3) RNA often occurs as both single- and partially double-stranded forms, whereas DNA most often occurs in a double-stranded form.

19. Although there are many types of RNA, the three main types described in this section are presented below:

ribosomal RNA: rRNA combines with proteins to form ribosomes that function to align mRNA and charged tRNA molecules during translation.

transfer RNA: tRNAs are involved in protein synthesis in that they represent a "link" between the sequences in DNA (as reflected in mRNA) and the ordering of amino acids in proteins. Transfer RNAs are specific in that each species is attached to only one type of amino acid.

messenger RNA: The coding sequence in DNA is transferred to the site of protein synthesis by a relatively short-lived molecule called messenger RNA. In eukaryotes, mRNA carries genetic information from the nucleus to the cytoplasm. It is the sequence of bases in mRNA that specifies the order of amino acids in proteins.

20. The nitrogenous bases of nucleic acids (nucleosides, nucleotides, and single- and double-stranded polynucleotides) absorb UV light maximally at wavelengths of 254 to 260 nm. Using this phenomenon, one can often determine the presence and concentration of nucleic acids in a mixture. Because proteins absorb UV light maximally at 280 nm, this is a relatively simple way of dealing with mixtures of biologically important molecules.

UV absorption is greater in single-stranded molecules (hyperchromic shift) than in double-stranded structures. Therefore, one can easily determine, by applying denaturing conditions, whether a nucleic acid is in the single- or double-stranded form. In addition, A-T rich DNA denatures more readily than G-C rich DNA. Therefore, one can estimate base content by denaturation kinetics.

21. Various treatments, such as heat, and certain chemical environments cause separation of the hydrogen bonds that hold together the complementary strands of DNA. Under these conditions, double-stranded DNA is changed to single-stranded DNA.

22. *A hyperchromic effect* is the increased absorption of UV light as double-stranded DNA (or RNA, for that matter) is converted to single-stranded DNA. As illustrated in the text, the change in absorption is quite significant, with a structure of higher G-C content *melting* at a higher temperature than an A-T rich nucleic acid. If one monitors the UV absorption with a spectrophotometer during the melting process, the hyperchromic shift can be observed. The T_m is the point on the profile (temperature) at which half (50 percent) of the sample is denatured.

23. Because G-C base pairs are formed with three hydrogen bonds whereas A-T base pairs by two such bonds, it takes more energy (higher temperature) to separate G-C pairs.

24. The reassociation of separate complementary strands of a nucleic acid, either DNA or RNA, is based on hydrogen bonds forming between A-T (or U) and G-C.

25. In one sentence of their first *Nature* paper, Watson and Crick state,

> It has not escaped our notice that the specific pairing we have postulated immediately suggests a possible copying mechanism for the genetic material.

The model itself indicates that unwinding of the helix and separation of the double-stranded structure into two single strands immediately expose the specific hydrogen bonds through which new bases are brought into place.

26. (1) As shown, the extra phosphate is not normally expected.

(2) In the adenine ring, a nitrogen is at position 8 rather than position 9.

(3) The bond from the C-1' to the sugar should form with the N at position 9 (N-9) of the adenine.

(4) The dinucleotide is a "deoxy" form; therefore, each C-2' should not have a hydroxyl group. Notice the hydroxyl group at C-2' on the sugar of the adenylic acid.

(5) At the C-5 position on the thymine residue, there should be a methyl group.

(6) There are too many bonds at the N-3 position on the thymine.

(7) There are too few bonds at the C-5 of thymine.

27. **(a)** The X-ray diffraction studies would indicate a helical structure, for it is on the basis of such data that a helical pattern is suggested. The fact that it is irregular may indicate different diameters (base pairings), additional strands in the helix, kinking, or bending.

(b) The hyperchromic shift would indicate considerable hydrogen bonding, possibly caused by base pairing.

(c) Such data may suggest irregular base pairing in which purines bind purines (all the bases presented are purines), thus giving the atypical dimensions.

(d) Because of the presence of ribose, the molecule may show more flexibility, kinking, and/or folding.

Although there are several situations possible for this model, the phosphates are still likely to be far apart (on the outside) because of their strong like charges. Hydrogen bonding probably exists on the inside of the molecule, and there is probably considerable flexibility, kinking, and/or bending.

28. Because cytosine pairs with guanine and uracil pairs with adenine, the result would be a base substitution of G:C to A:T after rounds of replication.

29. Under this condition, the hydrolyzed 5-methyl cytosine becomes thymine.

30. Without knowing the exact bonding characteristics of hypoxanthine or xanthine, it may be difficult to predict the likelihood of each pairing type. It is likely that both are of the same class (purine or pyrimidine) because the names of the molecules indicate a similarity. In addition, the diameter of the structure is constant, which, under the model to follow, would be expected. In fact, hypoxanthine and xanthine are both purines.

Because there are equal amounts of A, T, and H, one could suggest that they are hydrogen bonded to one another; the same may be said for C, G, and X. Given the molar equivalence of erythrose and phosphate, an alternating sugar-phosphate-sugar backbone as in "earth-type" DNA would be acceptable. A model of a triple helix would be acceptable, because the diameter is constant. Given the chemical similarities to "earth-type" DNA, it is probable that the unique creature's DNA follows the same structural plan.

31. (a) Heat application would yield a hyperchromic shift if the DNA is double-stranded. One could also get a rough estimation of the GC content from the kinetics of denaturation and the degree of sequence complexity from comparative renaturation studies.

(b) Determination of base content by hydrolysis and chromatography could be used for comparative purposes and could also provide evidence as to the strandedness of the DNA.

(c) Antibodies for Z-DNA could be used to determine the degree of left-handed structures, if present.

(d) Sequencing the DNA from both viruses would indicate sequence homology. In addition, through various electronic searches readily available on the Internet (*www.ncbi.nlm.nih.gov*, for example), one could determine whether similar sequences exist in other viruses or in other organisms.

32. The way the question is stated suggests that DNA that is separated electrophoretically is of the same shape (long rod). In fact, DNA can exist in a variety of shapes, as seen in supercoiled plasmids, relaxed (nicked) plasmids, and linear molecules. Size comparisons with DNA must be such that linear molecules are compared with linear molecules, supercoiled with supercoiled, and so on. In comparing DNA migration to RNA, even though RNA molecules have the same charge-to-mass ratios, they also exist in a variety of shapes. Complementary intrastrand base pairing can make more compact structures compared to the more relaxed, open conformation. For electrophoretic size comparisons, RNA molecules must be denatured to eliminate secondary structural variables.

33. One of the basic principles of gel electrophoresis is that shorter molecules migrate at a faster rate through a given gel than longer ones. Although a number of factors other than acrylamide concentration would be involved, depending on the length of the gel, it might be wise to use the 12 percent acrylamide recipe so that the short fragments will not reach the end of the gel and enter the buffer before the longer ones leave the wells.

Chapter 10: DNA Replication and Recombination

Concept Areas	Corresponding Problems
In Vitro Experiments	1, 2, 3, 4, 5, 6, 22, 26, 27
Eukaryotic Replication	14, 15, 16, 18, 25
Base Composition	8, 19
Enzymology	1, 7, 9, 10, 11, 12, 13, 15, 16, 17, 20, 21, 23
Telomerase	1, 24

Structures and Processes Checklist – Significant concepts that deserve special attention are identified with a "∗".

(check topic when mastered – provide examples where appropriate – understand the context of each entry)

- **Semiconservative Replication∗**
  - complementarity∗
  - hydrogen bonds∗
  - semiconservative replication∗
  - conservative replication∗
  - dispersive replication∗
  - Meselson–Stahl Experiment∗
  - $^{15}NH_4Cl$∗
  - ammonium chloride
  - heavy isotope
  - centrifugation∗
  - *E. coli*
  - gradient centrifugation∗
  - ^{15}N-DNA∗
  - "new" DNA
  - ^{14}N-DNA∗
  - "lighter band"∗
  - intermediate density∗

- $^{14}N/^{15}N$
  - replication in eukaryotes∗
  - Taylor, Woods, Hughes∗
  - *Vicia faba*
  - autoradiography∗
  - "grains"
  - radioactive thymidine∗
  - origin of replication
  - unidirectional∗
  - bidirectional∗
  - replication fork
  - replicon
  - *oriC*
  - *E. coli*
- **Five Polymerases∗**
  - DNA polymerase I∗
  - chain elongation
  - 3'-OH∗

94

- 5' to 3' direction*
- DNA polymerase II, III, IV, V*
- primer*
- repair enzymes
- holoenzyme
- core enzyme
- enzyme subunits
- replisome
- **Complex Issues***
  - RNA primer*
  - 9mers
  - 13mers
  - DnaA
  - DnaB
  - DnaC
  - single-stranded binding proteins
  - SSBPs
  - supercoiling
  - DNA gyrase
  - DNA topoisomerases
  - initiation of DNA synthesis*
  - continuous DNA synthesis
  - discontinuous synthesis*
  - antiparallel*
  - leading strand*
  - lagging strand*
  - 1000 to 2000 nucleotides
  - Okazaki fragments*
  - DNA ligase

- *lig*
- concurrent synthesis*
- processivity
- proofreading*
- **Coherent Model***
- **Replication Is Controlled***
  - conditional mutations*
  - temperature-sensitive mutation
- **DNA Replication***
  - initiation
  - ARSs*
  - consensus sequence*
  - prereplication complex
  - origin recognition complex
  - ORC
  - eukaryotic polymerases*
  - polymerase switching
  - replication through chromatin
  - chromatin assembly factors
  - CAFs
- **Ends of Linear Chromosomes***
  - telomeres
  - double-stranded breaks
  - DSBs
  - telomere structure*
  - G-quartets
  - *Tetrahymena*
  - replication at telomers*
  - telomerase

- 5'-TTGGGG-3'
- reverse transcription*
- **DNA Recombination***
  - general recombination
  - homologous recombination*

- heteroduplex DNA molecules*
- branch migration
- Holliday structure*
- RecA protein
- RecB, C, D proteins

F10-1 Shorthand structures for 3' and 5' nucleotides.

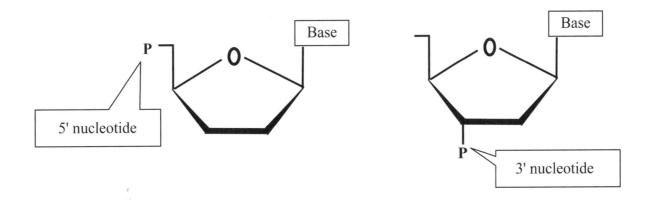

F10-2 Illustration of the influence of a conditional mutation on protein structure and function.

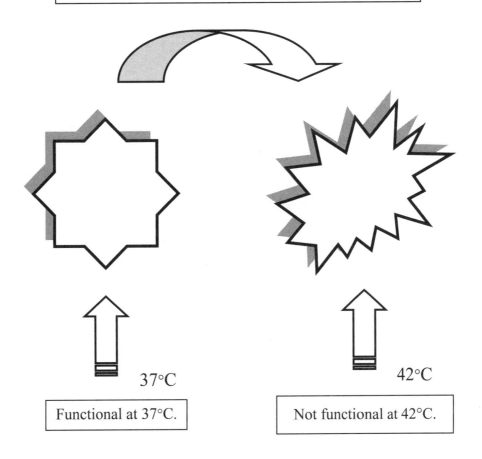

Changes in the environment of the protein may cause conformational changes in the protein to alter the function of that protein.

37°C

42°C

Functional at 37°C.

Not functional at 42°C.

F10-3 Figure relating to question 4 in the problems section depicts labeling pattern under *conservative* and *dispersive* replication patterns.

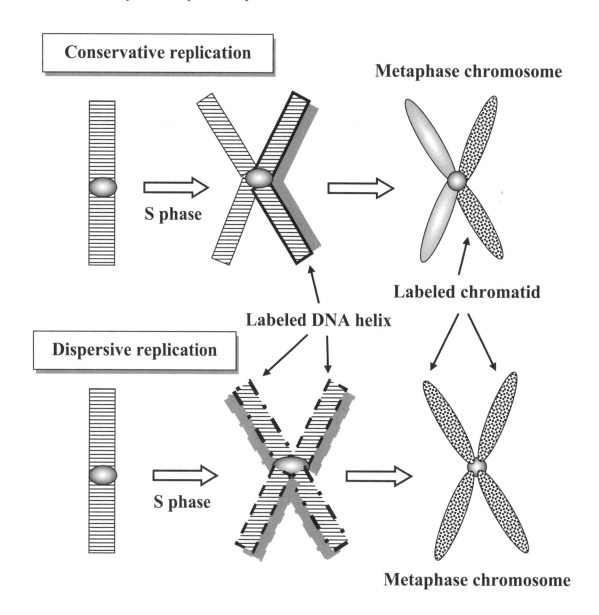

Answers to Now Solve This

10-1. Under a conservative scheme, the first round of replication in ^{14}N medium produces one "dense" double helix and one "light" double helix, in contrast to the "intermediate density" of the DNA in the semiconservative mode. Therefore, after one round of replication in the ^{14}N medium, the conservative scheme can be ruled out. After one round of replication in ^{14}N under a dispersive model, the DNA is of intermediate density, just as it is in the semiconservative model. However, in the next round of replication in ^{14}N medium, the density of the DNA is between the intermediate and "light" densities and therefore could be ruled out.

10-2. If the DNA contained parallel strands in the double helix and the polymerase were able to accommodate such parallel strands, there would be continuous synthesis and no Okazaki fragments. Several other possibilities exist. If the DNA strands were replicated as complete single strands, the synthesis could begin at the opposite free ends. In addition, if the DNA existed only as a single strand, the same results would occur.

1. (a) Two classic experiments, one using *E. coli* and the other using *Vicia faba,* demonstrated, using density and radioisotope labeling respectively, that replication is semiconservative in prokaryotes and eukaryotes. In both cases, daughter DNA molecules are each composed of one parental strand and one newly synthesized DNA strand.

(b) A mutant in DNA polymerase I (*polA1*) was nevertheless capable of synthesizing biologically active DNA, leading to the conclusion that at least one other enzyme is responsible for replicating DNA *in vivo.*

(c) *In vitro* studies by Kornberg and coworkers indicated that DNA strand elongation occurs by addition of nucleotides at the 3' end. During chain elongation, two of the outer phosphates of the precursor dNTP are cleaved and the remaining phosphate attaches to the 3'-OH group of the deoxyribose. *In vivo* or *in vitro*, DNA polymerases, including polymerase III, are capable only of 5' to 3' synthesis.

(d) Two lines of evidence indicated that DNA synthesis is discontinuous. First, in newly formed DNA, relatively short nucleotide fragments are hydrogen bonded to the template strands. Second, these short nucleotide fragments accumulate in ligase-deficient mutants of *E. coli.*

(e) Because eukaryotic chromosomes are linear rather than circular, free ends exist. It was predicted that such free ends would create the problem of shortening because of the 5'–3' nature of DNA synthesis and the inability of DNA polymerases to initiate synthesis without a free 3'-OH. The finding of the telomerase enzyme and a number of terminal repeats at the ends of chromosomes provided supported the prediction of chromosome shortening and its solution.

2. The differences among the three models of DNA replication relate to the manner in which the new strands of DNA are oriented as daughter DNA molecules are produced.

Conservative: In the conservative scheme, the original double helix remains as a complete unit and the new DNA double helix is produced as a single unit. The old DNA is completely conserved.

Semiconservative: In the semiconservative scheme, each daughter strand is composed of one old DNA strand and one new DNA strand. Separation of hydrogen bonds is required.

Dispersive: In the dispersive scheme, the original DNA strand is broken into pieces and the new DNA in the daughter strand is interspersed among the old pieces. Separation of the individual covalent phosphodiester bonds is required for this mode of replication.

3. The Meselson and Stahl experiment has the following components. By labeling the pool of nitrogenous bases of the DNA of *E. coli* with the heavy isotope ^{15}N, it was possible to "follow" the "old" DNA. This was accomplished by growing the cells for many generations in medium containing ^{15}N. Cells were transferred to ^{14}N medium so that "new" DNA could be detected. A comparison of the density of DNA samples at various times in the experiment (initial ^{15}N culture and subsequent cultures grown in the ^{14}N medium) showed that after one round of replication in the ^{14}N medium, the DNA was half as dense (intermediate) as the DNA from bacteria grown only in the ^{15}N medium. In a sample taken after two rounds of replication in the ^{14}N medium, half of the DNA was of the intermediate density and the other half was as dense as DNA containing only ^{14}N DNA.

4. Refer to the text for an illustration of the labeling of *Vicia* chromosomes under a Taylor, Woods, and Hughes experimental design. Notice that only those cells that pass through the S phase in the presence of the ^{3}H-thymidine are labeled and that each double helix (per chromatid) is "half-labeled." See F10-3 in this book for a graphic description of the conservative and dispersive replication patterns.

(a) Under a conservative scheme, all of the newly labeled DNA will go to one sister chromatid, whereas the other sister chromatid will remain unlabeled. In contrast to a semiconservative scheme, the first replicative round would produce one sister chromatid that has label on both strands of the double helix. (See F10-3 above.)

(b) Under a dispersive scheme, all of the newly labeled DNA will be interspersed with unlabeled DNA. Because these preparations (metaphase chromosomes) are highly coiled and condensed structures derived from the "spread-out" form at interphase (which includes the S phase), it is impossible to detect the areas where label is not found. Rather, both sister chromatids would appear as evenly labeled structures. (See F10-3 above.)

5. Because the semiconservative scheme predicts that *half* of the DNA in each daughter double helix is labeled, it would be difficult to envision a scheme in which three strands are replicated in such a semiconservative manner. It would seem that either the conservative or dispersive scheme would fit more appropriately. To examine the nature of replication, one could devise an experiment similar to that of Meselson and Stahl or Taylor, Woods, and Hughes.

6. The *in vitro* replication requires a DNA template, a primer to give a double-stranded portion, a divalent cation (Mg^{2+}), and all four of the deoxyribonucleoside triphosphates: dATP, dCTP, dTTP, and dGTP. The lowercase "d" refers to the deoxyribose sugar.

7. Prior to the development of highly efficient methods of enzyme isolation, large cultures, containing large numbers of bacterial cells, were needed to yield even small quantities of enzymes.

8. Several analytical approaches showed that the products of DNA polymerase I were probably copies of the template DNA. *Base composition* was used initially to compare both templates and products. Within experimental error, those data strongly suggested that the DNA replicated faithfully.

9. The *in vitro* rate of DNA synthesis using DNA polymerase I is slow, being more effective at replicating single-stranded DNA than double-stranded DNA. In addition, it is capable of degrading as well as synthesizing DNA. Such degradation suggested that it functioned as a repair enzyme. In addition, DeLucia and Cairns discovered a strain of *E. coli* (*pol*A1) that still replicated its DNA but was deficient in DNA polymerase I activity.

10. Each precursor (dNTP) to DNA synthesis is added to the 3' end of a growing chain by the removal of the terminal phosphates and the formation of a covalent bond. The 3'-OH provided by the 3' nucleotide directly participates in the formation of that covalent bond.

11. The *pol*AI mutation was instrumental in demonstrating that DNA polymerase I activity was not necessary for the *in vivo* replication of the *E. coli* chromosome. Such an observation opened the door

for the discovery of other enzymes involved in DNA replication.

12. All three enzymes share several properties. First, none can *initiate* DNA synthesis on a template but all can *elongate* an existing DNA strand, assuming there is a template strand as shown in the figure below. Polymerization of nucleotides occurs in the 5' to 3' direction; each 5' phosphate is added to the 3' end of the growing polynucleotide.

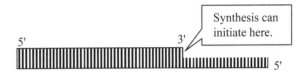

All three enzymes are large, complex proteins with a molecular weight in excess of 100,000 daltons, and each has 3' to 5' exonuclease activity. Refer to the text.

DNA polymerase I:
    Polymerization
    3'–5' exonuclease activity
    5'–3' exonuclease activity
    Present in large amounts
    Relatively stable
    Removal of RNA primer

DNA polymerase II:
    Polymerization
    3'–5' exonuclease activity
    Possibly involved in repair function

DNA polymerase III:
    Polymerization
    3'–5' exonuclease activity
    Essential for replication
    Complex molecule

13. Refer to the text for a listing of the components of DNA polymerase III. The active form of the enzyme is called the holoenzyme. The region responsible for actual polymerization is called the "core" portion.

14. Given a stretch of double-stranded DNA, one could initiate synthesis at a given point and replicate strands either in one direction only (unidirectional) or in both directions (bidirectional), as shown below. Notice that in the text, the synthesis of complementary strands occurs in a *continuous* 5'>3' mode on the leading strand in the direction of the replication fork, and in a *discontinuous* 5'>3' mode on the lagging strand opposite the direction of the replication fork. Such discontinuous replication forms Okazaki fragments.

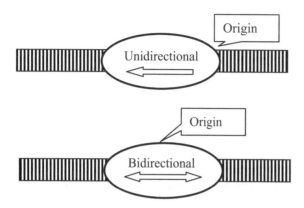

15. *Helicase, dna*A, and *single-stranded DNA binding proteins* initially unwind, open, and stabilize DNA at the initiation point. *DNA gyrase*, a DNA topoisomerase, relieves supercoiling generated by helix unwinding. This process involves breaking both strands of the DNA helix.

16. *Okazaki fragments* are relatively short DNA fragments (1000 to 2000 bases in prokaryotes) that are synthesized in a discontinuous fashion on the lagging strand during DNA replication. Such fragments appear to be necessary because template DNA is not available for 5'>3' synthesis until some degree of continuous DNA synthesis occurs on the leading strand in the direction of the replication fork. The isolation of such fragments provides support for the scheme of replication shown in the text. DNA *ligase* is required to form phosphodiester linkages in gaps that are generated when DNA polymerase I removes RNA primer and meets newly synthesized DNA ahead of it.

Notice in the text that the discontinuous DNA strands are ligated together into a single continuous strand. *Primer* RNA is formed by RNA primase to serve as an initiation point for the production of DNA strands on a DNA template. None of the DNA polymerases are capable of initiating synthesis without a free 3' hydroxyl group. The primer RNA provides that group and thus can be used by DNA polymerase III.

17. The synthesis of DNA is thought to follow the pattern described in the text. The model involves opening and stabilization of the DNA helix, priming DNA with synthesis with RNA primer, movement of replication forks in both directions, which includes

elongation of RNA primers in continuous and discontinuous 5'>3' modes, and their removal by the exonucleolytic activity of DNA polymerase I. Okazaki fragments generated in the replicative process are joined together with DNA ligase. DNA gyrase relieves supercoils generated by DNA unwinding.

18. Eukaryotic DNA is replicated in a manner that is very similar to that of *E. coli*. Synthesis is bidirectional, continuous on one strand and discontinuous on the other, and the requirements of synthesis (four deoxyribonucleoside triphosphates, divalent cation, template, and primer) are the same. Okazaki fragments of eukaryotes are about one-tenth the size of those in bacteria.

Because there is a much greater amount of DNA to be replicated and DNA replication is slower, there are multiple initiation sites for replication in eukaryotes (and increased DNA polymerase per cell) in contrast to the single replication origin in prokaryotes. Replication occurs at different sites during different intervals of the S phase. The proposed functions of four DNA polymerases are described in the text. Because most eukaryotic chromosomes are linear, enzymes such as telomerase are needed to replicate the telomeres, or ends of chromosomes.

19. Even though the base composition of two species may be similar, *sequences* can vary considerably.

20. (a) In *E. coli*, 100 kb are added to each growing chain per minute. Therefore, the chain should be about 4,000,000 bp.

(b) Given $(4 \times 10^6 \text{ bp}) \times 0.34 \text{ nm/bp} =$

$$1.36 \times 10^6 \text{ nm or } 1.3 \text{ mm}$$

21. (a) No repair from DNA polymerase I and/or DNA polymerase III.

(b) No DNA ligase activity.

(c) No primase activity.

(d) Only DNA polymerase I activity.

(e) No DNA gyrase activity.

22. First, ^{3}H-thymidine would be incorporated into newly synthesized DNA. Second, under denaturing centrifugation conditions, the short Okazaki fragments are free to form a distinct peak of lower molecular weight DNA in a centrifugation profile. Third, as time passes, the Okazaki fragments that are synthesized on the lagging strand are joined by DNA ligase so that larger strands are formed, which form their own higher molecular weight peak.

23. (a) Because DNA polymerase III is essential for DNA chain elongation, it is necessary for replication of the *E. coli* chromosome. Thus, strains that are mutant for this enzyme must contain conditional mutations or may rely on DNA polymerase I and replicate their DNA more slowly.

(b) The 3'–5' exonuclease activity is involved in proofreading. Thus, proofreading would be hampered in such mutant strains and a higher than expected mutation rate would occur.

24. Telomerase activity is present in germ-line tissue to maintain telomere length from one generation to the next. In other words, telomeres cannot shorten indefinitely without eventually eroding genetic information.

25. Because synthesis is bidirectional, one can multiply the rate of synthesis by 2 to come up with a figure of 18,000 bases replicated per 5 minutes (30 bases/second × 300 seconds). Dividing 1.6×10^8 by 1.8×10^4 gives 0.88×10^4, or about 8800 replication sites.

26. If replication is conservative, the first autoradiograms (see metaphase I in the text) would have label distributed on only one side (chromatid) of the metaphase chromosome, as follows:

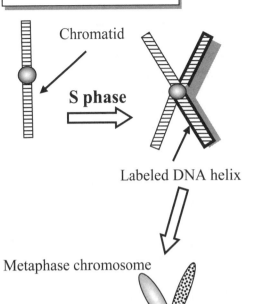

Conservative replication

Chromatid

S phase

Labeled DNA helix

Metaphase chromosome

Labeled chromatid

27. Conservative replication can be eliminated. Under a conservative mode of replication, both of the original DNA strands remain together in one chromatid and the two new strands form a single double helix in the other chromatid. Such is not the case in this figure.

Chapter 11: Chromosome Structure and DNA Sequence Organization

Concept Areas	Corresponding Problems
Viral and Bacterial Chromosomes	1, 2, 16, 17, 21
Mitochondrial and Chloroplast DNA	3
Specialized Chromosomes	1, 4, 5, 6
Organization of DNA in Chromatin	1, 7, 8, 9, 10, 11, 12, 18, 19
Organization of the Eukaryotic Genome	7, 12, 13, 14, 15, 20

Structures and Processes Checklist – Significant concepts that deserve special attention are identified with a "*".

(check topic when mastered – provide examples where appropriate – understand the context of each entry)

- **Chromosome Structure**
  - light microscopy
  - electron microscopy
  - chromatin structure

- **Viral and Bacterial Chromosomes***
  - DNA or RNA
  - linear or circular
  - single-stranded
  - double-stranded
  - φXI74
  - polyoma virus
  - bacteriophage lambda*
  - λ
  - nucleoid
  - T2
  - DNA-binding proteins
  - HU
  - H1

- **Mitochrondia and Chloroplasts***
  - mtDNA*
  - introns*
  - vertebrate mtDNA*
  - heavy (H)
  - light (L)
  - cpDNA*
  - fairly uniform
  - larger than mtDNA
  - introns*

- **Specialized Chromosomes***
  - polytene chromosomes*
  - chromomeres
  - puff*
  - lampbrush chromosomes*
  - chromomeres
  - first prophase of meiosis*

Chapter 11 Chromosome Structure and DNA Sequence Organization

- **DNA in Chromatin***
  - chromatin
  - nucleosome*
  - histones*
  - electron microscopy*
  - endonuclease digestion*
  - micrococcal nuclease
  - nucleosome core particle
  - H1
  - linker DNA
  - chromatin remodeling*
  - histone tails
  - acetylation*
  - methylation*
  - phosphorylation*
  - heterochromatin*
  - euchromatin*
  - position effect
  - chromosome banding*
  - G-banding
  - C-banding
- **Complex Sequence Organization***
  - repetitive DNA*
  - satellite DNA*
  - highly repetitive DNA*
  - molecular hybridization*
  - centromeric DNA*
- centromere*
  - CEN region
  - kinetochore*
  - alphoid family
  - telomeric DNA sequences*
  - telomere*
  - TERRA
  - middle repetitive sequences
  - VNTRs*
  - STRs*
  - minisatellites*
  - DNA fingerprinting*
  - microsatellites*
  - repetitive transposed sequences*
  - SINEs*
  - LINEs*
  - transposable sequences*
  - *Alu* family*
  - L1 family
  - retrotransposons*
  - multiple copy genes
  - ribosomal RNA
  - 5S rRNA
- **Few Functional Genes**
  - pseudogenes
  - reassociation kinetic analysis

Answers to Now Solve This

11-1. By having a circular chromosome, no free ends present the problem of linear chromosomes, namely, complete replication of terminal sequences.

11-2. Because eukaryotic chromosomes are "multirepliconic" in that there are multiple replication forks along their lengths, one would expect to see multiple clusters of radioactivity.

11-3. Volume of the nucleus = $(4/3)\pi r^3$

$= 4/3 \times 3.14 \times (5 \times 10^3 \text{nm})^3$

$= 5.23 \times 10^{11} \text{nm}^3$

Volume of the chromosome = $\pi r^2 \times \text{length}$

$= 3.14 \times 5.5\text{nm} \times 5.5\text{nm} \times (2 \times 10^9 \text{nm})$

$= 1.9 \times 10^{11} \text{nm}^3$

Therefore, the percentage of the volume of the nucleus occupied by the chromatin is

$1.9 \times 10^{11} \text{nm}^3 / 5.23 \times 10^{11} \text{nm}^3 \times 100 = \text{about } 36.3\%$

Chapter 11 Chromosome Structure and DNA Sequence Organization

Solutions to Problems and Discussion Questions

1. (a) Higher-level circular chromosomal structures and compositions have been revealed through both chemical and observational (microscopic) analyses.

(b) Using radioactively labeled RNA precursors followed by autoradiography, researchers discovered a high rate of RNA incorporation, indicating intense transcription.

(c) Early evidence came from endonuclease digestion that yielded DNA fragments of about 200 base pairs in length. Electron microscopic, X-ray and neutron-scattering observations revealed the structure of nucleosomes and their relationship to DNA.

(d) Base sequences and organizational motifs of satellite DNA are common to many regions within and flanking centromeric DNA. In humans, most satellite DNA is of the alphoid family found mainly in centromeric regions that total up to 3 million base pairs. In addition, *in situ* hybridization of satellite DNA clusters in heterochromatic regions flanking centromeres. Rapid renaturation of DNA also indicates the presence of repetitive sequences.

2. Bacteriophage λ has a linear, double-stranded DNA while in the phage coat and upon infection closes to form a circular chromosome with a size of about 50 kb. T2 phage also has a linear, double-stranded DNA chromosome of less than 200 kb. *E. coli* has a circular, double-stranded DNA chromosome of about 4.2×10^3 kb. Both intact phages are about 1/150 the size of *E. coli*. Because phages are obligate parasites of bacteria, they are dependent on their hosts for the manufacture of materials for their replication. Bacteria contain all genetic information for metabolism, replication, and *de novo* synthesis of numerous life-supporting materials. Phages, on the other hand, contain relatively few genes, namely, those needed to adsorb, inject, and produce progeny using primarily bacterial materials.

3. Mitochondrial DNA and chloroplast DNA exist as double-stranded closed circles that replicate semiconservatively. They are both free of chromosomal proteins that are characteristic of eukaryotic chromosomes. Lengths of mtDNA but not cpDNA vary, and multiple copies of each DNA may occur in each organelle. Few, if any, introns or repetitive sequences occur in mtDNA; however, cpDNA does contain duplications and long noncoding regions.

4. Polytene chromosomes are formed from numerous DNA replications, pairing of homologs, and absence of strand separation or cytoplasmic division. Each chromosome contains about 1000–5000 DNA strands in parallel register. They appear in specific tissues, such as salivary glands, of many dipterans such as *Drosophila*. They appear as comparatively long, wide fibers with sharp light and dark sections (bands) along their length. Such bands (chromomeres) are useful in chromosome identification and detection of chromosomal rearrangements.

5. Puffs represent active genes as evidenced by staining and uptake of labeled RNA precursors as assayed by autoradiography.

6. Lampbrush chromosomes are typically present in vertebrate oocytes and are so named because their appearance is similar to brushes used to clean kerosene lamp chimneys in the nineteenth century. They are also found in spermatocytes of some insects. They are found as diplotene stage structures and are active uncoiled versions of condensed meiotic chromosomes. Lampbrush chromosomes are typically viewed using light and electron microscopy.

7. Here, as greater DNA content per cell is associated with eukaryotes, one cannot universally equate genomic size with an increase in organismic complexity. There are numerous examples in which DNA content per cell varies considerably among closely related species. Because of the diverse cell types of multicellular eukaryotes, a variety of gene products are required, which may be related to the increase in DNA content per cell. In addition, the advantage of diploidy automatically increases DNA content per cell. However, looking at the question in another way, it is likely that a much higher *percentage* of the genome of a prokaryote is actually involved in phenotype production than in a eukaryote.

Eukaryotes have evolved the capacity to obtain and maintain what appear to be large amounts of "extra," perhaps "junk," DNA. This concept will be examined in subsequent chapters of the text. Prokaryotes, on the other hand, with their relatively short life cycle, are extremely efficient in their accumulation and use of their genome.

Given the larger amount of DNA per cell and the requirement that the DNA be partitioned in an orderly fashion to daughter cells during cell division, certain mechanisms and structures (mitosis, nucleosomes, centromeres, etc.) have evolved for packaging and distributing the DNA. In addition, the genome is divided into separate entities (chromosomes) to perhaps facilitate the partitioning process in mitosis and meiosis.

8. Digestion of chromatin with endonucleases, such as micrococcal nuclease, gives DNA fragments of approximately 200 base pairs or multiples of such segments. X-ray diffraction data indicated a regular spacing of DNA in chromatin. Regularly spaced bead-like structures (nucleosomes) were identified by electron microscopy.

9. Nucleosomes are octomeric structures of two molecules of each histone (H2A, H2B, H3, and H4) except H1. On the surface of the nucleosomes and complexed with linker DNA is histone H1. A 146-base-pair sequence of DNA wraps around the nucleosome.

10. As chromosome condensation occurs, a 300-Å fiber is formed. It appears to be composed of five or six nucleosomes coiled together. Such a structure is called a solenoid. These fibers form a series of loops that further condense into the chromatin fiber and are then coiled into chromosome arms making up each chromatid.

11. *Heterochromatin* is chromosomal material that stains deeply and remains condensed when other parts of chromosomes, euchromatin, are otherwise pale and less condensed. Heterochromatic regions replicate late in S phase and are relatively inactive in a genetic sense because there are few genes present, or if they are present, they are repressed. Telomeres and the areas adjacent to centromeres are composed of heterochromatin.

12. There are three main categories of repetitive sequences. Heterochromatin is located within centromeres and telomeres. There are two types of tandem repeats, long and short DNA sequences. Transposable sequences are varied in structure and size and are generally interspersed throughout the entire genome in eukaryotes. There are multiple species of repetitive sequences within each of the above-mentioned categories.

13. Satellite DNA is identified by sedimentation equilibrium centrifugation as one or more additional peaks that represent DNA of a slightly different density. Satellite DNA falls into the highly repetitive category and consists of relatively large numbers of

short sequences. Such sequences are clustered in heterochromatic areas typically flanking the centromere. Such areas are often void of typical euchromatic genes.

14. Long interspersed elements (LINEs) are repetitive transposable DNA sequences in humans. The most prominent family, designated **L1**, is about 6.4kb each and is represented about 100,000 times. LINEs are often referred to as retrotransposons because their mechanism of transposition resembles that used by retroviruses.

15. (a) Because there are 200 base pairs per nucleosome (as defined in this problem) and 10^9 base pairs, there would be 5×10^6 nucleosomes.

(b) Because there are 5×10^6 nucleosomes and nine histones (including H1) per nucleosome, there must be $9(5 \times 10^6)$ histone molecules: 4.5×10^7. **(c)** Because there are 10^9 base pairs present and each base pair is 3.4 Å, the overall length of the DNA is 3.4×10^9 Å. Dividing this value by the packing ratio (50) gives 6.8×10^7 Å .

16. The first step of this solution is to convert all of the given values to cubic Angstroms, remembering that 1 mm = 10,000 Å. Using the formula πr^2 for the area of a circle and $(4/3)\pi r^3$ for the volume of a sphere, the following calculations apply:

Volume of DNA: 3.14×10 Å $\times 10$ Å $\times$
$$(50 \times 10^4 \text{ Å}) = 1.57 \times 10^8 \text{ Å}^3$$

Volume of capsid: $4/3$ (3.14×400 Å $\times$
$$400 \text{ Å} \times 400 \text{ Å}) = 2.67 \times 10^8 \text{ Å}^3$$

Because the capsid head has a greater volume than the volume of DNA, the DNA will fit into the capsid.

17. One base pair occupies 0.34 nm; therefore, the equation would be as follows:

$52 \mu\text{m}/(0.34 \text{ nm/bp}) \times 1000 \text{ nm/mm} =$
$$152{,}941 \text{ base pairs}$$

18. The intimate relationships among histones, nucleosomes, and DNA in chromatin clearly account for structural remodeling of chromosomes as the cell cycle proceeds from interphase to metaphase. That nucleosomes are associated with chromatin during periods of gene activity raises the question of the possible roles they play in influencing not only chromosome structure but also gene function. The finding that natural chemical modification of nucleosomal components, as indicated in the question, increases gene activity suggests that changes in the binding of nucleosomes to DNA enable genes to be more accessible to factors that promote gene function. In addition, the finding that heterochromatin, containing fewer genes and more repressed genes, is undermethylated further supports the suggestion that histone modification is functionally related to changes in gene activity.

19. DNA replicates in a *semiconservative* fashion, with each daughter DNA double helix containing one new and one original single strand. Nucleosomes follow a *dispersive* pattern, with each daughter chromatid containing a mixture of old and original nucleosomes. One could test the distribution of nucleosomes by conducting an autoradiographic experiment similar to Taylor-Woods-Hughes, but instead of labeling the DNA with ^{3}H-thymidine, labeling some or all the histones H2A, H2B, H3, and H4 in nucleosomes.

20. Dividing 3×10^9 base pairs by 10^6 gives an average of 3000 base pairs or 3 kb between *Alu* sequences.

21. Bacteriophage lambda is composed of a double-stranded, linear DNA molecule of about 48,000 base pairs. It is capable of forming a closed, double-stranded circular molecule because of a 12-base-pair, single-stranded, complementary "overhanging" sequence at the 5′ end of each single strand.

Chapter 12: The Genetic Code and Transcription

Concept Areas	Corresponding Problems
Genetic Code	1, 2, 14, 23, 25
Deciphering the Code	1, 3, 6, 7, 9, 10, 11, 12, 22
Characteristics of the Code	1, 4, 5, 8, 12, 15, 16, 23, 25
Information Flow	1, 15, 17, 18, 19
RNA Structure	1, 13, 20, 21, 24

Structures and Processes Checklist – Significant concepts that deserve special attention are identified with a "∗".

(check topic when mastered – provide examples where appropriate – understand the context of each entry)

- **Genetic Code∗**
  - messenger RNA∗
  - mRNA∗
  - ribosomes
  - decoding∗
  - protein synthesis∗
- **Genetic Code Characteristics∗**
  - linear form
  - ribonucleotide sequence
  - complementarity∗
  - "word"
  - triplet code∗
  - unambiguous∗
  - degenerate∗
  - "start"
  - "stop"
  - initiate∗
  - terminate∗

- **Early Studies Established Code**
  - triplet nature∗
  - frameshift mutations∗
  - frame of reading∗
- **Nirenberg, Matthaei, Others∗**
  - *in vitro* (cell-free) system∗
  - polynucleotide phosphorylase∗
  - RNA homopolymers∗
  - mixed copolymers∗
  - RNA heteropolymers∗
  - mixed copolymer experiment∗
  - triplet binding assay∗
  - anticodon∗
  - triplet RNA-ribosome complex∗
  - degenerate
  - unambiguous
  - 64 triplets∗
  - repeating copolymers∗

- termination codons*
- **Coding Dictionary***
  - 61 amino acid assignments*
  - 3 terminating triplets*
  - pattern of degeneracy
  - wobble hypothesis*
  - 30-40 tRNA species*
  - ordered genetic code
  - initiation
  - termination
  - N-formylmethionine*
  - fmet*
  - initiator codons
  - termination codons
  - UAG, UAA, UGA*
  - nonsense mutation*
- **Genetic Code Confirmed***
  - bacteriophage MS2
  - colinearity*
- **Nearly Universal Code***
  - mtDNA*
  - exceptions to the code
- **Overlapping Genes***
  - different initiation points*
- **Transcription of RNA from DNA***
  - transcription*
  - information flow*
- **RNA Polymerase***
  - *n*(NTP)

- *n*(PP$_i$)
- (NMP)n
- holoenzyme*
- σ
- sigma factor*
- promoters*
- template strand*
- partner strand*
- template binding
- transcription start site*
- consensus sequences*
- Pribnow box*
- TATAAT*
- *cis*-acting elements*
- *trans*-acting factors*
- TATA box*
- initiation
- chain elongation*
- DNA/RNA duplex
- 5'–3' extension*
- hairpin secondary structure
- termination factor
- ρ
- rho
- polycistronic mRNA*
- cistron*
- monocistronic mRNA*
- **Transcription in Eukaryotes***
  - chromatin remodeling*

- transcription factors*
- TFs
- enhancers*
- silencers*
- RNA processing*
- pre-mRNA
- heterogeneous nuclear RNA*
- hnRNA
- hnRNPs*
- split genes*
- splicing
- initiation of transcription
- RNA polymerase II*
- RNP II
- proximal-promoter elements*
- enhancers
- silencers
- Golberg-Hogness box*
- TATA box*

- **Heterogeneous Nuclear RNA***
  - caps and tails*
  - posttranscriptional modification*

- 7-methyl guanosine*
- 7-mG
- methyl group*
- CH₃
- 3' poly-A*
- AAUAAA

- **Coding Regions Interrupted***
  - intron*
  - intervening sequence*
  - exon*
  - ovalbumin gene*
  - collagen*
  - 50 introns
  - dystrophin*
  - self-splicing RNAs
  - ribozymes*
  - transesterification reactions
  - spliceosome*
  - isoforms*

- **Visualized by Microscopy**
  - *Xenopus laevis*
  - rDNA

F12-1 Illustration of the processes, transcription and translation, involved in protein synthesis. Such relationships are often called the central dogma.

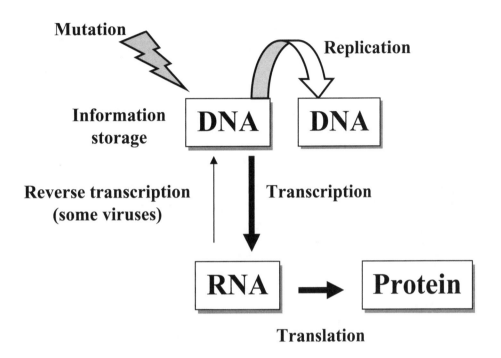

F12-2 Illustration of transcription in prokaryotes coupled with translation. Transcription involves production of RNA from a DNA template.

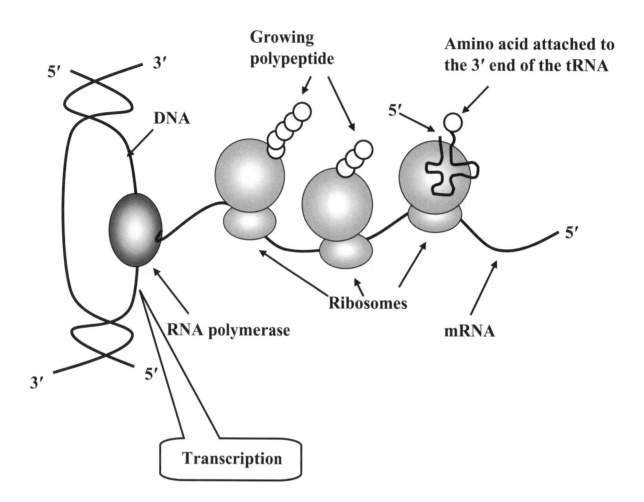

Answers to Now Solve This

12-1. (a) The way to determine the fraction of each triplet that will occur with a random incorporation system is to determine the likelihood that each base will occur in each position of the codon (first, second, third), then multiply the individual probabilities (fractions) for a final probability (fraction).

GGG	=	$3/4 \times 3/4 \times 3/4$	=	27/64
GGC	=	$3/4 \times 3/4 \times 1/4$	=	9/64
GCG	=	$3/4 \times 1/4 \times 3/4$	=	9/64
CGG	=	$1/4 \times 3/4 \times 3/4$	=	9/64
CCG	=	$1/4 \times 1/4 \times 3/4$	=	3/64
CGC	=	$1/4 \times 3/4 \times 1/4$	=	3/64
GCC	=	$3/4 \times 1/4 \times 1/4$	=	3/64
CCC	=	$1/4 \times 1/4 \times 1/4$	=	1/64

(b) Glycine:

GGG and one G_2C (adds up to 36/64)

Alanine:

one G_2C and one C_2G (adds up to 12/64)

Arginine:

one G_2C and one C_2G (adds up to 12/64)

Proline:

one C_2G and CCC (adds up to 4/64)

(c) With the wobble hypothesis, variation can occur in the third position of each codon. Below are possible unordered codon assignments:

Glycine:	GGG, GGC
Alanine:	CGG, GCC, CGC, GCG
Arginine:	GCG, GCC, CGC, CGG
Proline:	CCC,CCG

12-2. Assume that you have introduced a copolymer (ACACACAC...) to a cell-free protein synthesizing system. There are two possibilities for establishing the reading frames: ACA if one starts at the first base and CAC if one starts at the second base. These would code for two different amino acids (ACA = threonine; CAC = histidine) and would produce repeating polypeptides that would alternate *thr-his-thr-his*... or *his-thr-his-thr*....

Because of a triplet code, a trinucleotide sequence will, once initiated, remain in the same reading frame and produce the same code all along the sequence regardless of the initiation site.

Given the sequence CUACUACUACUA, notice the different reading frames producing three different sequences, each containing the same amino acid:

Codons:	CUA	CUA	CUA	CUA...
Amino Acids:	leu	leu	leu	leu...
	UAC	UAC	UAC	UAC...
	tyr	tyr	tyr	tyr...
	ACU	ACU	ACU	ACU...
	thr	thr	thr	thr...

If a tetranucleotide is used, such as ACGUACGUACGU...:

Codons:	ACG	UAC	GUA	CGU	ACG
Amino Acids:	thr	tyr	val	arg	thr
	CGU	ACG	UAC	GUA	CGU
	arg	thr	tyr	val	arg
	GUA	CGU	ACG	UAC	GUA
	val	arg	thr	tyr	val
	UAC	GUA	CGU	ACG	UAC
	tyr	val	arg	thr	tyr

Notice that the sequences are the same except that the starting amino acid changes.

12-3. Apply complementary bases, substituting U for T:

(a) Sequence 1: 3′-GAAAAAACGGUA-5′
Sequence 2: 3′-UGUAGUUAUUGA-5′
Sequence 3: 3′-AUGUUCCCAAGA-5′

(b) Sequence 1: *met-ala-lys-lys*
Sequence 2: *ser-tyr-[ter]*
Sequence 3: *arg-thr-leu-val*

(c) Apply complementary bases:

3′-GAAAAAACGGTA-5′

Chapter 12 The Genetic Code and Transcription

Solutions to Problems and Discussion Questions

1. (a) An initial understanding about the composition (unordered) of codons came from homopolymer and heteropolymer RNAs introduced into an *in vitro* system. Assays of the relative amino acid composition of resulting polypeptides indicated the composition of the bases in codons, but not their actual sequence.

(b) The specific sequences of the triplet codes were determined by the triplet binding assay and repeating copolymers of known sequence. When added to a cell-free system, a direct analysis of codon assignments was possible.

(c) Because the complete sequence of the RNA phage MS2 was known, scientists matched that sequence with protein products of MS2, which supported the code as derived from previous studies.

(d) Work with *E. coli* infected with phage showed that the synthesis of proteins was under the direction of newly synthesized RNA. Others were able to show that newly synthesized RNA formed during a phage infection of bacteria would hybridize only with phage DNA, thus demonstrating the dependence of RNA on the template nature of DNA.

(e) The most direct evidence for the presence of noncoding sequences in RNA and therefore the presence of split genes comes from hybridization experiments. When mature mRNAs are hybridized to DNA containing the genes specifying that mRNA, heteroduplexes form, indicating that sequences in the DNA are not always represented in mRNA products. In addition, studies that compare the sequences of DNAs to their corresponding RNAs and proteins show that DNA often contains sequences that are not represented in RNA and protein products.

2. In eukaryotes, protein synthesis occurs primarily in the cytoplasm, far from the location of DNA and the encoded information. In addition, whereas some of the basic amino acids would be able to associate directly with DNA, the acidic amino acids would be unable to do so. Thus, some sort of "adaptor" system was needed for DNA to direct amino acid assembly.

3. (a) The reason that (+++) or (– – –) restored the reading frame is that the code is triplet. By having the (+++) or (– – –), the translation system is "out of phase" until the third "+" or "–" is encountered. If the code contained six nucleotides (a sextuplet code),

then the translation system is "out of phase" until the sixth "+" or "–" is encountered. In this case, the "out of phase" region would probably be more extensive and likely cause more amino acid alterations, but the reading frame would eventually be established.

(b) Given a sextuplet code, restoration of the reading frames would occur only with the addition or loss of six nucleotides. Lay out a sequence such as

CATDOGPIGOWLCATDOGPIGOWLCAT...

and test parts "a" and "b" in the problem.

4. The UUACUUACUUAC tetranucleotide sequence will produce the following triplets depending on the initiation point: UUA = leu, UAC = tyr, ACU = thr, CUU = leu. Notice that because of the degenerate code, two codons correspond to the amino acid leucine.

The UAUCUAUCUAUC tetranucleotide sequence will produce the following triplets depending on the initiation point: UAU = tyr, AUC = ile, UCU = ser, CUA = leu. Notice that in this case, degeneracy is not revealed and all the codons produce unique amino acids.

5. From the repeating polymer ACACA..., one can say that threonine is either CAC or ACA. From the polymer CAACAA... with ACACA..., ACA is the only codon in common. Therefore, threonine would have the codon ACA.

6. As in the previous problem, the procedure is to find those sequences that are the same for the first two bases but that vary in the third base. Given that AGG = arg, information from the AG copolymer indicates that AGA also codes for arg and GAG must therefore code for glu.

Coupling this information with that of the AAG copolymer, GAA must also code for glu, and AAG must code for lys.

7. The basis of the technique is that if a trinucleotide contains bases (a codon) that are complementary to the anticodon of a charged tRNA, a relatively large complex is formed that contains the ribosome, the tRNA, and the trinucleotide. This complex is trapped in the filter, whereas the components by themselves are not trapped. If the amino acid on a charged, trapped tRNA is radioactive, then the filter becomes radioactive.

8. List the substitutions, then from the code table apply the codons to the original amino acids. Select codons that provide single base changes.

Original		Substitutions
threonine	- - - - - >	*alanine*
<u>AC</u> (U, C, A, or G)		<u>GC</u> (U, C, A, or G)
glycine	- - - - - >	*serine*
<u>GG</u> (U or C)		<u>AG</u> (U or C)
isoleucine	- - - - - >	*valine*
<u>AU</u> (U, C or A)		<u>GU</u> (U, C or A)

9. Apply the most conservative pathway of change.

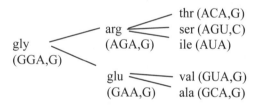

10. The enzyme generally functions in the degradation of RNA; however, in an *in vitro* environment, with high concentrations of the ribonucleoside diphosphates, the direction of the reaction can be forced toward polymerization. *In vivo*, the concentration of ribonucleoside diphosphates is low and the degradative process is favored.

11. Because poly U is complementary to poly A, double-stranded structures will be formed. In order for an RNA to serve as a messenger RNA, it must be single-stranded, thereby exposing the bases for interaction with ribosomal subunits and tRNAs.

12. Applying the coding dictionary, the following sequences are "decoded":

Sequence 1: met-pro-asp-tyr-ser-(term)

Sequence 2: met-pro-asp-(term)

The 12th base (a uracil) is deleted from sequence #1, thereby causing a frameshift mutation that introduced a terminating triplet UAA.

13. (a)

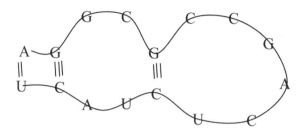

(b) 3′-TCCGCGGCTGAGATGA-5′ (use complementary bases, substituting T for U)

(c) 3′-GCU-5′

(d) Assuming that the AGG... is the first codon in the reading frame of the mRNA, the sequence would be

arg-arg-arg-leu-tyr

14. Given the sequence GGA, by changing each of the bases to the remaining three bases and then checking the code table, one can determine whether amino acid substitutions will occur.

G G A gly		G G U gly
U G A **term**		G G C gly
C G A **arg**		G G A gly
A G A **arg**		G G G gly
G U A **val**		U G U **cys**
G C A **ala**		C G U **arg**
G A A **glu**		A G U **ser**
G G U gly		G U U **val**
G G C gly		G C U **ala**
G G A gly		G A U **asp**

15. (a) Starting from the 5′ end and locating the AUG triplets, one finds two initiation sites leading to the following two sequences:

met-his-thr-tyr-glu-thr-leu-gly

met-arg-pro-leu-asp (or glu)

(b) In the shorter of the two reading sequences (the one using the internal AUG triplet), a UGA triplet was introduced at the second codon. Although not in the reading frames of the longer polypeptide (using the first AUG codon), the UGA triplet terminates the product starting at the second initiation codon.

16. By examining the coding dictionary, one will notice that the number of codons for each particular amino acid (synonyms) is directly related to the frequency of amino acid incorporation stated in the problem.

17. The central dogma of molecular genetics and, to some extent, all of biology states that DNA produces, through transcription, RNA, much of which (mRNA) is "decoded" (during translation) to produce proteins. See F12-2 for a graphic description.

18. RNA polymerase from *E. coli* is a complex, large (almost 500,000 daltons) molecule composed of subunits (α, β, β', σ) in the proportion $\alpha2$, β, β', σ for the holoenzyme. The β subunit provides catalytic function, whereas the sigma (σ) subunit is involved in recognition of specific promoters. The core enzyme is the protein without the sigma.

19. Ribonucleoside triphosphates and a DNA template in the presence of RNA polymerase and a divalent cation (Mg^{2+}) produce a ribonucleoside monophosphate polymer, DNA, and pyrophospate (diphosphate). Equimolar amounts of precursor ribonucleoside triphosphates and product ribonucleoside monophosphates and pyrophosphates (disphosphates) are formed. In *E. coli,* transcription and translation can occur simultaneously. Ribosomes attach to the 5' end of the nascent mRNA and progress to the 3' end during translation. Although transcription/translation can be "visualized" in *E. coli* (F12-2), the predominant components "visualized" are the strings of ribosomes (polysomes).

20. Whereas some folding (from complementary base pairing) may occur with mRNA molecules, they generally exist as single-stranded structures that are quite labile. Eukaryotic mRNAs are generally processed such that the 5' end is "capped" and the 3' end has a considerable string of adenine bases. It is thought that these features protect the mRNAs from degradation. Such stability of eukaryotic mRNAs probably evolved with the differentiation of nuclear and cytoplasmic functions. Because prokaryotic cells exist in a more unstable environment (nutritionally and physically, for example) than many cells of multicellular organisms, rapid genetic response to environmental change is likely to be adaptive. To accomplish such rapid responses, a labile gene product (mRNA) is advantageous. A pancreatic cell, which is developmentally stable and existing in a relatively stable environment, could produce more insulin on stable mRNAs for a given transcriptional rate.

21. It is likely that 3'-polyadenylation influences the overall configuration of RNA transcripts that then either by itself or in conjunction with proteins or other RNAs impacts the longevity of the transcript. Especially in eukaryotes, 3'-polyadenylation may also influence the transport of RNAs to and from cellular organelles. In addition, 3'-polyadenylation may facilitate or inhibit the association of RNAs to other cellular components, such as proteins, lipids, or nucleic acids.

22. First, compute the frequency (percentages would be easiest to compare) for each of the random codons.

For 4/5 C: 1/5 A:

CCC $= 4/5 \times 4/5 \times 4/5 = 64/125$ (51.2%)

$C_2A = 3(4/5 \times 4/5 \times 1/5) = 48/125$ (38.4%)

$CA_2 = 3(4/5 \times 1/5 \times 1/5) = 12/125$ (9.6%)

AAA $= 1/5 \times 1/5 \times 1/5 = 1/125$ (0.8%)

For 4/5 A: 1/5 C:

AAA $= 4/5 \times 4/5 \times 4/5 = 64/125$ (51.2%)

$A_2C = 3(4/5 \times 4/5 \times 1/5) = 48/125$ (38.4%)

$AC_2 = 3(4/5 \times 1/5 \times 1/5) = 12/125$ (9.6%)

CCC $= 1/5 \times 1/5 \times 1/5 = 1/125$ (0.8%)

Proline:	C_3 and one of the C_2A triplets
Histidine:	one of the C_2A triplets
Threonine:	one C_2A triplet and one A_2C triplet
Glutamine:	one of the A_2C triplets
Asparagine:	one of the A_2C triplets
Lysine:	A_3

23.

(a) #1: *nonsense mutation*
#2: *missense mutation*
#3: *frameshift mutation*

(b) #1: mutation in third position to A or G
#2: change U to C in third triplet
#3: removal of a G in the UGG triplet (trp)

(c) termination

(d) All of the amino acids can be assigned specific triplets including the third base of each triplet. Compare the sequences for the wild type and mutant #2. After removal of a G in the UUG triplet of tryptophan, the frameshift mutation shifts the first base of the following triplet to the third (often ambiguous) base of the previous triplet. The only tricky solution is with serine, which has six triplet possibilities, but it can still be resolved.

AUG UGG UAU CGU GGU AGU CCA ACA

(e) The mutation may be in a promoter or enhancer, although many posttranscriptional alterations are possible.

24. (a, b) Alternative splicing occurs when pre-mRNAs are spliced in more than one way to yield various combinations of exons in the final mRNA product. Upon translation of a group of alternatively spliced mRNAs, a series of related proteins, called isoforms, are produced. It is likely that alternative splicing evolved to provide a variety of functionally related proteins in a particular tissue from one original source. In other words, varieties of similar proteins can be produced by alternative splicing rather than independent evolution.

Some tissues might be more prone to develop alternative splicing if they depend on a number of related protein functions. In addition, if genes found in certain tissues have more exons in their active genes, alternative splicing would be expected. Although some information is available concerning the mechanisms of alternative splicing, at this time little is known about the underlying forces that drove the evolution of tissue-specific alternative splicing. The use of alternative splicing to generate varieties of products is also known to exist at different developmental stages. In such cases, as development occurs, different splicing mechanisms occur.

25. (a, b) Use the code table to determine the number of triplets that code each amino acid; then construct a graph and plot such as the one that follows:

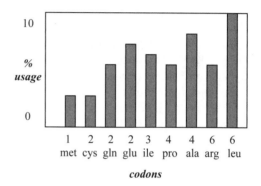

(c) There appears to be a weak correlation between the relative frequency of amino acid usage and the number of triplets for each.

(d) To continue to investigate this issue, one might examine additional amino acids in a similar manner. In addition, different phylogenetic groups use code synonyms differently. It may be possible to find situations in which the relationships are more extreme. One might also examine more proteins to determine whether such a weak correlation is stronger with different proteins.

Chapter 13: Translation and Proteins

Concept Areas	Corresponding Problems
Translation/Colinearity	5, 14
RNAs	1, 2, 3, 4, 7, 8, 13
Punctuation/Code	1, 6, 18
One-gene:One-enzyme	9
Pathways	1, 19, 20, 21
Proteins	1, 10, 11, 12, 15, 16, 17
Antibiotic Resistance	22

Structures and Processes Checklist – Significant concepts that deserve special attention are identified with a "*".

(check topic when mastered – provide examples where appropriate – understand the context of each entry)

- **Translation of mRNA***

  - transfer RNA*

  - tRNA

  - adaptor hypothesis*

  - anticodon*

  - ribosome structure*

  - rRNA

  - ribosomal proteins

  - monosome

  - Svedberg coefficient

  - 70S, 50S, 30S

  - 80S, 60S, 40S

  - 23S, 5S

  - 28S, 5.8S, 5S

  - 16S

  - 18S

  - associated proteins

- rRNA genes

- tRNA structure*

- 75–90 nucleotides

- symbolism of tRNAs*

- posttranscriptional modifications

- cloverleaf model of tRNA

- 3' to 5' direction

- anticodon loop

- 3' end pCpCpA

- 5'-Gp

- charging tRNA*

- aminoacyl tRNA synthetases*

- isoaccepting tRNAs*

- **Steps in Translation***

  - initiation*

  - initiation factors (IFs)

  - formylmethionine*

- fmet
- AUG*
- Shine-Dalgarno sequence
- initiation complex*
- elongation
- P (peptidyl) site
- A (aminoacyl) site
- peptidyl transferase*
- ribozyme*
- E (exit) site*
- elongation factors (EFs)
- termination*
- stop codons
- termination codons
- nonsense codons
- GTP-dependent release factors
- polyribosomes
- polysomes
- **High-Resolution Studies***
  - X-ray diffraction
  - crystallographic analysis
  - cryo-electron microscopy
- **Translation in Eukaryotes***
  - core sequence
  - expansion sequences
  - 7-methylguanosine
  - 7-mG
  - Kozak sequence
  - tRNA$_i^{Met*}$

- **Inborn Errors of Metabolism***
  - alkaptonuria
  - consanguine
- **One-Gene:One-Enzyme***
  - *Neurospora* mutants*
  - mimimal medium
  - nutritional mutation*
- **Human Hemoglobin***
  - one-gene:one-protein*
  - one-gene:one-polypeptide chain*
  - sickle-cell anemia*
  - sickle-cell trait
  - HbA
  - HbS
  - inherited molecular disease
- **Protein Structure***
  - polypeptide*
  - protein*
  - carboxyl group
  - amino group
  - R (radical) group*
  - side chain
  - central carbon (C) atom
  - nonpolar*
  - hydrophobic*
  - polar*
  - hydrophilic*
  - positively charged
  - negatively charged

- peptide bond*
- dipeptide
- tripeptide
- primary structure*
- secondary structure*
- α helix
- β-pleated sheet
- tertiary structure*
- quaternary structure*
- protein folding*
- protein misfolding*
- conformation*
- chaperone*
- heat-shock proteins*
- ubiquitin*
- proteasome
- scrapie*
- bovine spongioform encephalopathy

- mad cow disease*
- Creutzfeldt-Jacob disease*
- prions*
- Huntington disease*
- Alzheimer disease*
- Parkinson disease*
- **Proteins and Diverse Functions***
  - hemoglobin
  - myoglobin
  - collagen
  - keratin
  - actin
  - mioson
  - tubulin
  - immunoglobulins
  - transport proteins
  - histones
  - transcription factors
  - protein domains

F13-1 Polarity constraints associated with simultaneous transcription and translation in prokaryotes. The RNA polymerase is moving downward (arrow) in this sketch.

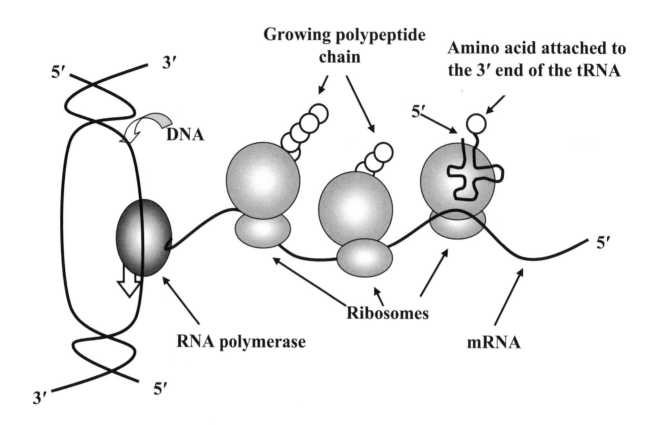

Answers to Now Solve This

13-1. One can conclude that the tRNA and not the amino acid is involved in recognition of the codon.

13-2. With the codes for valine being GUU, GUC, GUA, and GUG, single base changes from glutamic acid's GAA and GAG can cause the glu>>>val switch. The same can be said for lysine with its AAG codon. The normal glutamic acid is a negatively charged amino acid, whereas valine carries no net charge and lysine is positively charged. Given these significant charge changes, one would predict some, if not considerable, influence on protein structure and function. Such changes could stem from internal changes in folding or interactions with other molecules in the RBC, especially other hemoglobin molecules.

Chapter 13 Translation and Proteins

Solutions to Problems and Discussion Questions

1. (a) The base sequences in tRNA suggested a cloverleaf secondary structure due to within-strand complementary base pairing. Such a model was later supported by X-ray crystallography and denaturation studies.

(b) When UAA, UGA, or UAG triplets occur at internal sites in genes, premature translation termination occurs and verifies the chain terminating function of these triplets.

(c) Examination of nutritional mutations in *Neurospora* showed that upsets in metabolic pathways could result from mutant genes that segregated and assorted in typical fashion. In some cases, sufficient information was available to show that defective enzymes caused the metabolic upset. Thus, mutant genes must be responsible for the production of defective enzymes.

(d) Because enzymes are proteins, it is reasonable to conclude that genes make proteins. In addition, early work on hemoglobin showed that one gene was responsible for making one of the polypeptide chains in hemoglobin.

2. A functional polyribosome will contain the following components: mRNA, charged tRNA, large and small ribosomal subunits, elongation and perhaps initiation factors, peptidyl transferase, GTP, Mg^{2+}, nascent proteins, and possibly GTP-dependent release factors.

3. Transfer RNAs are "adaptor" molecules in that they provide a way for amino acids to interact with sequences of bases in nucleic acids. Amino acids are specifically and individually attached to the 3' end of tRNAs that possess a three-base sequence (the anticodon) to base-pair with three bases of mRNA. Messenger RNA, on the other hand, contains a copy of the triplet codes that are stored in DNA. The sequences of bases in mRNA interact, three at a time, with the anticodons of tRNAs.

Enzymes involved in transcription include the following: RNA polymerase (*E. coli*) and RNA polymerase I, II, III (eukaryotes). Those involved in translation include the following: aminoacyl tRNA synthetases, peptidyl, and transferase.

4. It was reasoned that there would not be sufficient affinity between amino acids and nucleic acids to account for protein synthesis. For example, acidic amino acids would not be attracted to nucleic acids.

With an adaptor molecule, specific hydrogen bonding could occur between nucleic acids, and specific covalent bonding could occur between an amino acid and a nucleic acid tRNA.

5. The sequence of base triplets in mRNA constitutes the sequence of codons. A three-base portion of the tRNA constitutes the anticodon.

6. Because three nucleotides code for each amino acid, there would be 423 code letters (nucleotides), 426 including a termination codon. This assumes that other features such as the poly-A tail, the 5' cap, promoter, and 5' and 3' untranslated sequences are omitted.

7. The steps involved in tRNA charging are outlined in the text. An amino acid in the presence of ATP, Mg^{2+}, and a specific aminoacyl synthetase produces an amino acid–AMP enzyme complex (+ PP$_i$). This complex interacts with a specific tRNA to produce the aminoacyl tRNA.

8. The four sites in tRNA that provide for specific recognition are the following: attachment of the specific amino acid, interaction with the aminoacyl tRNA synthetase, interaction with the ribosome, and interaction with the codon (anticodon).

9. Because enzymes are a subclass of the general term *protein*, a *one-gene:one-protein* statement might seem to be more appropriate. However, some proteins are made up of subunits, each different type of subunit (polypeptide chain) being under the control of a different gene. Under this circumstance, the *one-gene:one-polypeptide* statement might be more reasonable.

It turns out that many functions of cells and organisms are controlled by stretches of DNA that either produce no protein product (operator and promoter regions, for example) or have more than one function, as in the case of overlapping genes and alternative mRNA splicing. A simple statement regarding the relationship of a stretch of DNA to its physical product is difficult to justify.

10. The quaternary level results from the associations of individual polypeptide chains.

11. Sickle-cell anemia is coined a *molecular* disease because it is well understood at the molecular level, at the level of a base change in DNA that leads to an amino acid change in the β chain of hemoglobin. It is a *genetic* disease in that it is inherited from one generation to the next. It is not contagious, as might be the case of a disease caused by a microorganism. Diseases caused by microorganisms may not necessarily follow family blood lines, whereas genetic diseases do.

12. A person who has the sickle cell gene in the heterozygous state is a carrier. A person who is homozygous for the sickle cell gene has sickle-cell anemia. A single base change occurs at the sixth amino acid position in the β chain of hemoglobin. Such a change causes the incorporation of valine instead of glutamic acid. As a result of this change, both the structure and function of the hemoglobin molecule are altered.

13. Dividing 20 by 0.34 gives the number of nucleotides (about 59) occupied by a ribosome. Dividing 59 by 3 gives the approximate number of triplet codes, approximately 20.

14. "Fine-mapping," meaning precise mapping of mutations *within* a gene, is possible in some phage systems because many recombinants can often be generated relatively easily. Having the precise intragenic location of mutations as well as the ability to isolate the products, especially mutant products, allows scientists to compare the locations of lesions within genes.

Mutations occurring nearer the initiation site in a gene will produce proteins with defects near the N-terminus. In this problem, the lesions cause chain termination; therefore, the nearer the mutations to the 5' end of the mRNA, the shorter the polypeptide product. Relating the position of the mutation with the length of the product establishes the colinear relationship.

15. As stated in the text, the four levels of protein structure are the following:

Primary: the linear arrangement or sequence of amino acids. This sequence determines the higher-level structures.

Secondary: α-helix and β-pleated sheet structures generated by hydrogen bonds between components of the peptide bond.

Tertiary: folding that occurs as a result of interactions of the amino acid side chains. These interactions include, but are not limited to, the following: covalent disulfide bonds between cysteine residues, interactions

of hydrophilic side chains with water, and interactions of hydrophobic side chains with each other.

Quaternary: the association of two (dimer) or more polypeptide chains. Called *oligomeric*, such a protein is made up of more than one protein.

Because all higher levels are dependent on the sequence of amino acids (primary structure), it is the primary structure that is most influential in determining protein structure and function.

16. There are probably as many different types of proteins as there are different types of structures and functions in living systems. Some examples follow:

Oxygen transport: hemoglobin, myoglobin
Structural: collagen, keratin, histones
Contractile: actin, myosin
Immune system: immunoglobins
Cross-membrane transport: a variety of proteins in
    and around membranes, such as receptor proteins
Regulatory: hormones, perhaps histones

17. Enzymes function to regulate catabolic and anabolic activities of cells. They influence (lower) the *energy of activation,* thus allowing chemical reactions to occur under conditions that are compatible with living systems. Enzymes possess active sites and/or other domains that are sensitive to the environment. The active site is considered to be a crevice, or pit, that binds reactants, thus enhancing their interaction. The other domains mentioned above may influence the conformation and therefore function of the active site.

18. All of the substitutions involve one base change.

19. Even though three gene pairs are involved, notice that because of the pattern of mutations, each cross may be treated as monohybrid **(a)** or dihybrid **(b, c)**.

(a) F_1:   *AABbCC* = speckled

  F_2: 3   *AAB_CC* = speckled
     1   *AAbbCC* = yellow

(b) F_1:   *AABbCc* = speckled

  F_2: 9   *AAB_C_* = speckled
     3   *AAB_cc* = green
     3   *AAbbC_* = yellow ⎱
     1   *AAbbcc* = yellow ⎰ 4

(c) F_1:   *AaBBCc* = speckled

  F_2: 9   *A_BBC_* = speckled
     3   *A_BBcc* = green
     3   *aaBBC_* = colorless ⎱ 4
     1   *aaBBcc* = colorless ⎰

20. Because cross **(a)** is essentially a monohybrid cross, there would be no difference in the results if crossing over occurred (or did not occur) between the *a* and *b* loci.

21. The best way to approach these types of problems, especially when the data are organized in the form given, is to realize that the substance (supplement) that "repairs" a strain, as indicated by a (+), is *after* the metabolic block for that strain. In addition, and most important, the substance that "repairs" the highest number of strains either is *the end product* or is *closest to the end product*.

Looking at the table, notice that the supplement tryptophan "repairs" all the strains. Therefore, it must be at the end of the pathway or at least after all the metabolic blocks (defined by each mutation). Indole "repairs" the next highest number of strains (3); therefore, it must be second from the end. Indole glycerol phosphate "repairs" two of the four strains, so it is third from the end. Anthranilic acid "repairs" the least number of strains, so it must be early (first) in the pathway.

Minimal medium is void of supplements, and mutant strains involving this pathway would not be expected to grow (or be "repaired"). The pathway therefore would be as follows:

AA----->IGP----->I----->TRY

To assign the various mutations to the pathway, keep in mind that if a supplement "repairs" a given mutant, the supplement must be after the metabolic block. Applying this rationale to the above pathway, the metabolic blocks are created at the following locations:

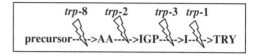

trp-8   trp-2   trp-3 trp-1

precursor--⚡->AA---⚡->IGP--⚡->I--⚡->TRY

22.

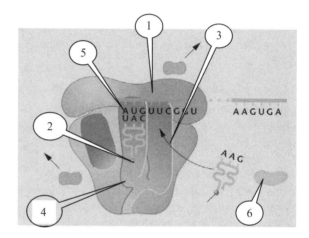

Chapter 14: Gene Mutation, DNA Repair, and Transposition

Concept Areas	Corresponding Problems
Classes of Mutations	1, 3, 4, 6, 11
Detection of Mutations	2, 15, 17
Spontaneous Mutation Rates	8
Induced Mutations	1, 9, 10, 11
Molecular Basis of Mutation	4, 5, 6, 19, 20, 21, 22, 23, 24, 29
Conditional Mutations	7
Repair of DNA	1, 12, 13, 18
UV Radiation and Skin Cancer	14, 16, 25
High-Energy Radiation	14
Transposable Elements	26, 27, 28

Structures and Processes Checklist – Significant concepts that deserve special attention are identified with a "*".

(check topic when mastered – provide examples where appropriate – understand the context of each entry)

- **Classification of Mutations***
  - spontaneous*
  - induced*
  - cosmic sources
  - mineral sources
  - mutation rate*
  - somatic mutations*
  - germ-line mutations*
  - autosomal mutations*
  - X-linked mutations*
  - homogametic female
  - point mutation*
  - base substitution*
  - missense mutation*
  - nonsense mutation*
  - silent mutation*
  - transition
  - transversion
  - frameshift mutation*
  - loss-of-function*
  - null mutations*
  - gain-of-function*
  - visible mutation
  - nutritional mutation*
  - biochemical mutation
  - behavioral mutation
  - regulatory mutation*
  - lethal mutation
  - conditional mutation*
  - temperature-sensitive mutation

- neutral mutation*
- replication errors*
- tautomers*
- replication slippage
- tautomeric shifts*
- depurination*
- deamination*
- oxidative damage
- reactive oxidants*
- **Induced Mutations***
  - base analogs*
  - 5-bromouracil
  - 5-BU
  - bromodeoxyuridine
  - BrdU
  - 2-amino purine
  - 2-AP
  - ultraviolet radiation*
  - UV
  - electromagnetic spectrum
  - pyrimidine dimers*
  - ionizing radiation*
  - X rays
  - gamma rays
  - cosmic rays
  - free radicals*
- **Single-Gene Mutations***
  - approximately 20,000 genes
  - splicing mutations*

- trinucleotide repeat sequences*
- **DNA Repair Systems***
  - proofreading*
  - mismatch repair*
  - DNA polymerase III*
  - DNA methylation*
  - adenine methylase*
  - endonuclease*
  - exonuclease*
  - postreplication repair*
  - SOS repair*
  - photoreactivation repair*
  - UV damage*
  - photoreactivation enzyme*
  - thymine dimers*
  - excision repair*
  - base excision repair*
  - BER
  - DNA glycosylase*
  - apyrimidinic site*
  - apurinic site*
  - AP endonuclease*
  - nucleotide excision repair*
  - NER
  - xeroderma pigmentosum*
  - XP
  - UV-induced lesions
  - unscheduled DNA synthesis*
  - somatic cell hybridization*

- ○ heterokaryon*
- ○ complementation*
- ○ double-stranded break repair*
- ○ DSB repair
- ○ homologous recombination repair*
- ○ nonhomologous end joining
- ○ Ames test*
- ○ **Transposable Elements***
  - ○ transposons*
  - ○ insertion sequences*
  - ○ IS elements
  - ○ transposase*
  - ○ inverted terminal repeats
  - ○ ITRs
  - ○ Tn elements*
  - ○ R factors*
  - ○ Ac-Ds system*
- ○ *dissociation*
- ○ *Ds*
- ○ *activator*
- ○ *Ac*
- ○ mobile controlling elements*
- ○ *Copia**
- ○ *P* elements*
- ○ *Drosophila*
- ○ direct terminal repeat
- ○ DTR
- ○ hybrid dysgenesis*
- ○ germ-line transformation*
- ○ LINES*
- ○ SINES*
- ○ *Alu* element*
- ○ evolutionary implications*
- ○ recombinase

F14-1 Graphic representation of the relationship between mutation and Darwinian evolutionary theory. Mutation provides the original source of variation on which natural selection operates.

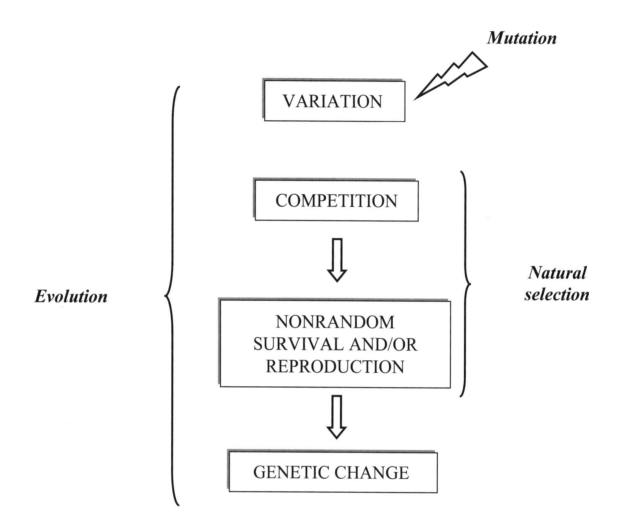

F14-2 Illustration of the difference between somatic and germ-line mutations. Somatic mutations are not passed to the next generation, whereas those in the germ line may be passed to offspring.

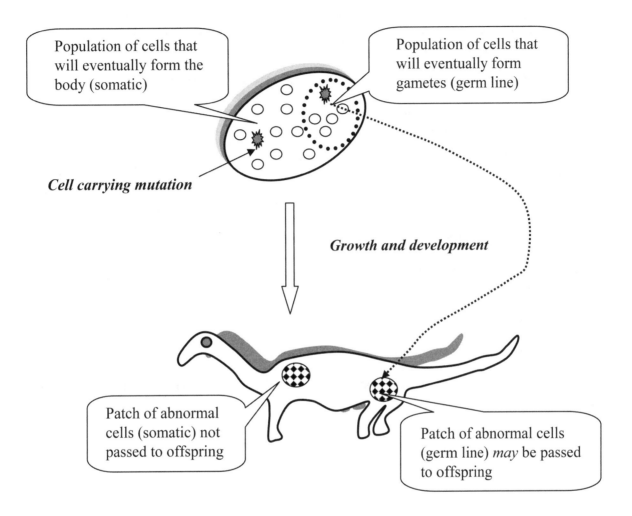

Answers to Now Solve This

14-1. The phenotypic influence of any base change is dependent on a number of factors, including its location in coding or non-coding regions, its potential in dominance or recessiveness, and its interaction with other base sequences in the genome. If a base change is located in a non-coding region, there may be no influence on the phenotype; however, some non-coding regions in a traditional sense may influence other genes and/or gene products. If a mutation occurring in a coding region acts as a full recessive, there should be no influence on the phenotype. If the mutant gene acts as a dominant, then there would be an influence on the phenotype. Some genes interact with other genes in a variety of ways that would be difficult to predict without additional information.

14-2. There are several ways in which an unexpected mutant gene may enter a pedigree. If a gene is incompletely penetrant, it may be present in a population and only express itself under certain conditions. It is unlikely that the gene for hemophilia behaved in this manner. If a gene's expression is suppressed by another mutation in an individual, it is possible that offspring may inherit a given gene and not inherit its suppressor. Such offspring would have hemophila. Because all genetic variations must arise at some point, it is possible that the mutation in Queen Victoria's family was new, arising in a cell of the father. Lastly, it is possible that the mother was heterozygous and by chance, no other individuals in her family were unlucky enough to receive the mutant gene.

14-3. Any agent that inhibits DNA replication, either directly or indirectly, through mutation and/or DNA crosslinking, will suppress the cell cycle and may be useful in cancer therapy. Because guanine alkylation often leads to mismatched bases, such bases can often be repaired by a variety of mismatched repair mechanisms. However, DNA crosslinking can be repaired by recombinational mechanisms; thus, for such agents to be successful in cancer therapy, suppressors of DNA repair systems are often used in conjunction with certain cancer drugs. See Wang, Z. et al. 2001. J Nat'l Cancer Inst. 93(19):1434-6.

14-4. Ethylmethane sulfonate (EMS) alkylates the keto groups at the sixth position of guanine and at the fourth position of thymine. In each case, base-pairing affinities are altered and transition mutations result. Altered bases are not readily repaired and once the transition to normal bases occurs through replication, such mutations avoid repair altogether.

Solutions to Problems and Discussion Questions

1. (a) When no known agents are involved and a mutation occurs and there is no indication of a mutation in the "family line," that mutation is considered to have arisen spontaneously.

(b) Numerous studies, beginning with those of Muller (1927) and Stadler (1928), showed that the occurrence of mutations could be associated with X rays. Since that time, various chemicals and radiation have been tested by a number of screening strategies. When the frequency of mutation in a test organism increases in concert with exposure to a given agent, that agent is classified as a mutagen.

(c) In addition to postreplication, SOS, photo-reactivation, and excision repair, various proofreading functions have been discovered in polymerases. Each has provided evidence that many mutations, once generated, may trigger repair.

2. Mutations are the "windows" through which geneticists look at the normal function of genes, cells, and organisms. When a mutation occurs, it allows the investigator to formulate questions as to the function of the normal allele of that mutation. For example, hemophilia is an inherited blood-clotting disease. Because there are three different inherited forms of the disease, two X-linked and one autosomal, all determined by nonallelic genes, one can say that there are at least three different proteins involved in blood clotting. At a different level, mutations provide "markers" with which biologists can study the genetics and dynamics of populations.

3. When conducting genetic screens, one assumes that all the cells of an organism are genetically identical. Therefore, the organism responds to the screen, enabling detection of the mutation. If a somatic cell of a multicellular organism is mutated, it is highly unlikely that the organism will be sufficiently altered to respond to a screen. That's not to say that somatic mutations can't influence the organism. Cancer cells generally originate from a single altered cell and can have a profound influence on the fate of an organism.

4. It is true that *most* mutations are thought to be deleterious to an organism. A gene is a product of perhaps a billion or so years of evolution, and it is only natural to suspect that random changes will probably yield negative results. However, *all* mutations may not be deleterious. Those few, rare variations that are beneficial will provide a basis for possible differential propagation of the variation. Such changes in gene frequency represent the basis of the evolutionary process. See F14-1 in this book.

5. As stated in the previous answer, a functional sequence of nucleotides, a gene, is likely to be the product of perhaps a billion or so years of evolution. Each gene and its product function in an environment that has also evolved, or co-evolved. A coordinated output of each gene product is required for life. Deviations from the norm, caused by mutation, are likely to be disruptive because of the complex and interactive environment in which each gene product must function. However, on occasion a beneficial variation occurs.

6. A diploid organism possesses at least two copies of each gene (except for "hemizygous" genes), and in most cases, the amount of product from one gene of each pair is sufficient for production of a normal phenotype. Recall that the condition of "recessive" is defined by the phenotype of the heterozygote. If output from one normal (nonmutant) gene in a heterozygote gives the same phenotype as in the normal homozygote, where there are two normal genes, the normal allele is considered "dominant."

	Phenotype, if mutant is	
<u>Genotypes</u>	<u>recessive</u>	<u>dominant</u>
wild/wild	wild	wild
wild/mutant	wild	mutant
mutant/mutant	mutant	mutant

7. A *conditional* mutation is one that produces a wild-type phenotype under one environmental condition and a mutant phenotype under a different condition. A conditional *lethal* is a gene that under one environmental condition leads to premature death of the organism.

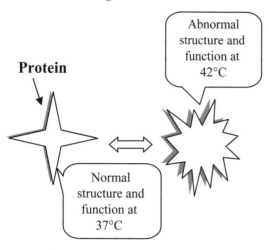

Protein

Abnormal structure and function at 42°C

Normal structure and function at 37°C

8. Watson and Crick recognized that various tautomeric forms, caused by single proton shifts, could exist for the nitrogenous bases of DNA. Such shifts could result in mutations by allowing hydrogen bonding of normally noncomplementary bases so that incorrect nucleotide bases may be added during DNA replication. As stated in the text, important tautomers involve keto-enol pairs for thymine and guanine and amino-imino pairs for cytosine and adenine.

9. All three of the agents are mutagenic because they cause base substitutions. Deaminating agents oxidatively deaminate bases such that cytosine is converted to uracil and adenine is converted to hypoxanthine. Uracil pairs with adenine and hypoxanthine pairs with cytosine. Alkylating agents donate an alkyl group to the amino or keto groups of nucleotides, thus altering base-pairing affinities. 6-ethyl guanine acts like adenine, thus pairing with thymine. Base analogs such as 5-bromouracil and 2-amino purine are incorporated as thymine and adenine, respectively, yet they base-pair with guanine and cytosine, respectively.

10. Frameshift mutations are likely to change more than one amino acid in a protein product because as the reading frame is shifted, a different set of codons is generated. In addition, there is the possibility that a nonsense triplet could be introduced, thus causing premature chain termination. If a single pyrimidine or purine has been substituted, then only one amino acid is influenced.

11. X rays are of higher energy and shorter wavelength than UV light. They have greater penetrating ability and can create more disruption of DNA.

12. When DNA is damaged, mutations are likely. In many cases, such mutations are deleterious to the health of the organism. Several mechanisms have evolved to reduce the impact of such mutations: cell-cycle arrest to quarantine a cell line or allow DNA repair and programmed cell death (apoptosis). If damaged DNA cannot be repaired through cell-cycle arrest, programmed cell death is often activated to rid the cell population of mutant cell lines.

13. *Photoreactivation* can lead to repair of UV-induced damage. An enzyme, photoreactivation enzyme, will absorb a photon of light to cleave thymine dimers. *Excision repair* involves the products of several genes, DNA polymerase I and DNA ligase, to clip out the UV-induced dimer, fill in, and join the phosphodiester backbone in the resulting gap. The excision repair process can be activated by damage that distorts the DNA helix. *Recombinational repair* is a system that responds to DNA that has escaped other repair mechanisms at the time of replication. If a gap is created on one of the newly synthesized strands, a "rescue operation" or "SOS response" allows the gap to be filled. Many different gene products are involved in this repair process: *rec*A and *lex*A. In SOS repair, the proofreading by DNA polymerase III is suppressed, and this therefore is called an "error-prone system."

14. Because mammography involves the use of X rays and X rays are known to be mutagenic, it has been suggested that frequent mammograms may do harm. This subject is presently under considerable debate. According to the International Agency for Research and Cancer (2008), breast cancer mortality can be reduced by 20 to 30 percent in women over 50 years of age when screening coverage is over 70 percent of the female population.

15. In the *Ames assay,* the compound to be tested is incubated with a mammalian liver extract to simulate an *in vivo* environment. This solution is then placed on culture plates with an indicator microorganism, *Salmonella typhimurium*, which is defective in its normal repair processes. The frequency of mutations in the tester strains is an indication of the mutagenicity of the compound. Because cancer results from the mutation of genes in somatic cells, mutagenic chemicals are considered to be potentially carcinogenic.

16. *Xeroderma pigmentosum* is a form of human skin cancer caused by perhaps several rare autosomal genes, which interfere with the repair of damaged

DNA. Studies with heterokaryons provided evidence for complementation, indicating that there may be as many as seven different genes involved. The enzymes responsible for nucleotide excision repair appear to be involved. Because cancer is caused by mutations in several types of genes, interfering with DNA repair can enhance the occurrence of these types of mutations.

17. Given that the cells were treated and then allowed to complete one round of replication, the final computation of the mutation rate should be divided by two (two cells are plated for each cell treated). The general expression for the mutation rate is the number of mutant cells divided by the total number of cells. In this case, the equation is as follows:

$$\frac{18 \times 10^1}{6 \times 10^7}$$

or 3×10^{-6}

Dividing by two (as stated above) gives

1.5×10^{-6}

18. Any condition that causes mutations in genes or DNA repair systems is likely to increase the rate of cancer. Specifically, mismatch repair defects are common in hereditary nonpolypopsis colon cancer; leukemias; lymphomas; and tumors of the ovary, prostate, and endometrium. The link between mutant mismatch repair systems and cancer is seen in mice engineered to have defects in mismatch repair genes. Such mice are cancer-prone.

19. There are numerous regions upstream from coding regions in a gene that are sensitive to mutation. Many mutations upset the regions that signal transcription factor and/or polymerase binding, thereby influencing transcription. Mutations within introns may affect intron splicing or other factors that determine mRNA stability or translation.

20. Replication slippage is a process that generates small deletions and insertions during DNA replication. Although it can occur anywhere in the genome, it is most prevalent in regions already containing repeated sequences. Thus, repeated sequences are hypermutable.

21. In some cases, chromosome breakage occurs that has significant influence on gene function. In other cases, deletions may occur that also influence gene function.

22. Unscheduled DNA synthesis represents DNA repair. One can determine complementation groupings by placing each heterokaryon giving a "–" into one group and those giving a "+" into a separate group. For instance, *XP1* and *XP2* are placed into the same group because they do not complement each other. However, *XP1* and *XP5* do complement ("+"); therefore, they are in different groups. Completing such pairings allows one to determine the following groupings:

XP1	*XP4*	*XP5*
XP2		*XP6*
XP3		*XP7*

The groupings (complementation groups) indicate that there are at least three "genes" that form products necessary for unscheduled DNA synthesis. All of the cell lines that are in the same complementation group are defective in the same product.

23. The cystic fibrosis gene produces a complex membrane transport protein that contains several major domains: a highly conserved ATP binding domain, two hydrophobic domains, and a large cytoplasmic domain, which probably serves in a regulatory capacity. The protein is like many ATP-dependent transport systems, some of which have been well studied. When a mutation causes clinical symptoms, fluid secretion is decreased and dehydrated mucus accumulates in the lungs and air passages. Mutations that radically alter the structure of the protein (frameshift, splicing, nonsense, deletions, duplications, etc.) would probably have more influence on protein function than those that cause relatively minor amino acid substitutions, although this generalization does not always hold true. A protein with multiple functional domains would be expected to react to mutational insult in a variety of ways.

24. (a) For those organisms that generate energy by aerobic respiration, a process occurs that involves the reduction of molecular oxygen. Partially reduced species are produced as intermediates and by-products of such molecular action: O_2^-, H_2O_2, and OH^- These species are potent electrophilic oxidants that escape mitochondria and attack numerous cellular components. Collectively, these are called reactive oxygen species (ROS).

(b)

oxoGuanine

Cytosine   Guanine

When casually examining the structures in the above diagrams, it is not immediately obvious that oxoG:A pairs should occur. However, hydrogen bonding can occur to any other base, including self pairs. Homopurine (A:A, G:G) and heteropurine (A:G) pairs represent anomalous base pairing possibilities, even with nonaltered bases. Whereas G:C is undoubtedly the most stable, several mispairs are actually stronger than the A:T pair.

Base pairing is complicated by the fact that the purines possess two H-bonding faces: the Watson-Crick face, involving ring positions 1 and 6 for adenine and 1, 2, and 6 for guanine, and the Hoogsteen face, involving ring positions 6 and 7. The typical pairing mode is indicated as *wc* where pairing occurs on the Watson-Crick face in the normal orientation, even for the mispair A:G. Alteration of pairing and favoring of the Hoogsteen face can be favored with the alteration generated by oxoGuanine. Indeed, triple helix configurations commonly involve the Hoogsteen face.

(c) If not repaired, the first round of replication involves the pairing of oxoG to adenine (see above), whereas in the next round of replication, adenine pairs with its normal thymine. Therefore, if one starts with a G:C pair, one ends up with an A:T pair.

(d) It turns out that G:G>T:A transversions are quite commonly found in human cancers and are especially prevalent in the tumor suppressor gene *p53*. Thus, the cellular defense system has been extensively studied. One component is a triphosphatase that cleanses the nucleotide precursor pool by removing the two outermost phosphates from oxo-dGTP. Another involves a DNA glycosylase that initiates repair of misreplicated oxoG:A by hydrolyzing the glycosidic bond linking the adenine base to the sugar. Another is a DNA gycosylase/lyase system that recognizes oxoG opposite cytosine. Of the three systems, the DNA glycosylases are probably the most effective.

25. (a,b) Individuals with xeroderma pigmentosum (XP) are much more likely to contract skin cancer in youth than non-XP individuals. By age 20, approximately 80 percent of the XP population has skin cancer compared with approximately 4 percent in the non-XP group. XP individuals lack one or more functional genes involved in DNA repair.

26. It is probable that the IS occupied or interrupted normal function of a controlling region related to the *galactose* genes, which are in an operon with one controlling upstream element.

27. Transposons cause changes in DNA in a variety of ways including massive chromosomal alterations. In most cases, changes in DNA are harmful to organisms, whereas in rare cases, an evolutionary advantage occurs because the new genetic variation confers a selective advantage.

28. First, although less likely, one might suggest that transposons, for one reason or another, are more likely to insert in noncoding regions of the genome. One might also suggest that they are more stable in such regions. Second, and more likely, it is possible that transposons insert rather randomly and that selection eliminates those that have interrupted coding regions of the genome. Because such regions are more likely to influence the phenotype, selection is more likely to influence such regions.

29. A hypothesis might be that of two forms of muscular dystrophy, one form, DMD, causes a more radical change in the dystrophin protein. In fact, DMD mutations are most commonly caused by changes in the reading frame of the dystrophin gene or situations that lead to premature termination of translation. The majority of BMD mutations are caused by gene rearrangements and point mutations that may alter an internal sequence of the dystrophin transcript and protein, but leave the reading frame intact.

Chapter 15: Regulation of Gene Expression

Concept Areas	Corresponding Problems
Overview	1, 2, 4, 5, 13, 18, 21, 24
Lactose Metabolism in E. coli	1, 6, 7, 8, 11
Positive and Negative Control	3, 4, 9, 14
Catabolite Repression	9, 11, 12
Transcription Initiation	10, 17, 20
Tryptophan Operon	5, 13
Model Systems	1, 2, 13, 14, 15, 16, 19, 24
Eukaryotic Regulation	1, 5, 21, 22, 23, 25, 26, 27

Structures and Processes Checklist – Significant concepts that deserve special attention are identified with a "∗".

(check topic when mastered – provide examples where appropriate – understand the context of each entry)

- o **Regulation of Gene Expression∗**
  - o activation∗
  - o repression∗
  - o *cis*-acting∗
  - o *trans*-acting∗
- o **Prokaryotic Gene Regulation∗**
  - o external conditions
  - o internal conditions
  - o inducible∗
  - o inducer∗
  - o constitutive∗
  - o repressible∗
  - o negative control∗
  - o positive control∗
- o **Lactose Metabolism in *E. coli*∗**
  - o *cis*-acting∗

- o *trans*-acting∗
- o structural genes
- o β–galactosidase∗
- o permease∗
- o transacetylase
- o regulatory mutations
- o gratuitous inducer∗
- o isopropylthiogalactoside
- o IPTG∗
- o constitutive mutants∗
- o repressor gene∗
- o operator region∗
- o operon model∗
- o negative control∗
- o repressor molecule∗
- o allosteric∗

- merozygote
- I^+
- I^-
- I^s
- O^+
- O^c
- isolation of the repressor*
- **Catabolite-Activating Protein***
  - CAP*
  - catabolite repression
  - cyclic adenosine monophosphate*
  - cAMP*
  - adenyl cyclase*
  - cooperative binding
  - CAP-cAMP*
- **Tryptophan Operon in *E. coli****
  - tryptophan synthase*
  - tryptophan*
  - corepressor*
  - leader sequence*
- **RNA Secondary Structure***
  - attenuation*
  - attenuator*
  - terminator*
  - antiterminator hairpin*
  - UGG triplets*
  - riboswitches*
  - 5'-untranslated region*
  - important domains

- default conformation*
- ligand
- ligand-binding site
- **Eukaryotic Gene Regulation***
- **Chromatin Modifications***
  - chromosome territories*
  - interchromosomal domains*
  - transcription factory*
  - RNA polymerase II
  - histone modifications*
  - nucleosomal chromatin remodeling*
  - histone acetyltransferase enzymes
  - HATs*
  - histone deacetylases
  - HDACs*
  - DNA methylation*
  - 5-azacytidine
- **Eukaryotic Transcription***
  - *cis*-acting sites
  - promoters*
  - promoter domains*
  - core promoter
  - proximal promoter elements*
  - focused promoters*
  - disperse promoters*
  - CG-rich regions
  - CAAT box*
  - CCAAT box
  - GC box*

- enhancer*
- tissue specific*
- silencer*
- activators and repressors*
- transcription factors*
- human metallothionein IIA
- *hMTIIA**

- **Transcription Factors***
  - general transcription factors
  - pre-initiation complex*
  - PIC*
  - elongation complex*
  - interactions*

- **Posttranscriptional Regulation***
  - alternative splicing*
  - *CT/CGRP* gene*
  - proteome
  - about 20,000 genes*
  - myotonic dystrophy*
  - *DMPK* gene
  - *ZNF9* gene
  - spliceopathies*
  - mRNA stability*

- steady-state level of mRNA*
- half-life
- adenosine-uracil rich element
- ARE*

- **Translational Controls***
  - p53 protein
  - Mdm2
  - ubiquitin

- **RNA-Induced Gene Silencing***
  - RNA interference*
  - RNAi*
  - small interfering RNAs
  - siRNAs*
  - microRNAs
  - miRNAs*
  - Dicer
  - RNA-induced silencing
  - RISC*
  - RITS*
  - single-gene defects*
  - viral infections*
  - molecular medicine

F15-1 Illustration of general processes of *negative* and *positive* control. If *negative* control is operating, the regulatory protein inhibits transcription. With *positive* control, transcription is stimulated.

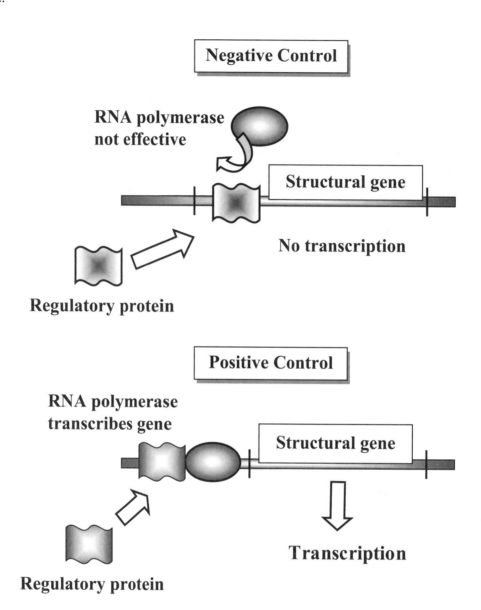

F15-2 Illustration of the nature of the product of the *I* gene. It can act "at a distance" because it is a protein that can diffuse through the cytoplasm and thus act in *trans*. There is no protein product of the operator gene; therefore, it can act only in *cis*.

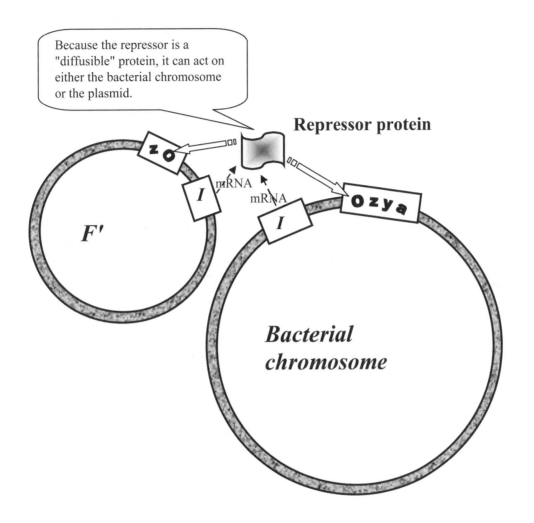

Chapter 15 Regulation of Gene Expression

Answers to Now Solve This

15-1. (a) Because of the deletion of a base early in the *lac Z* gene, there will be "frameshift" of all the reading frames downstream from the deletion, thereby altering many amino acids. It is likely that either premature chain termination of translation will occur (from the introduction of a nonsense triplet in a reading frame) or the normal chain termination will be ignored. Regardless, a mutant condition for the *Z* gene will be likely. If such a cell is placed on a lactose medium, it will be incapable of growth because β-galactosidase is not available. **(b)** If the deletion occurs early in the *A* gene, one might expect impaired function of the *A* gene product, but it will not influence the use of lactose as a carbon source.

15-2. In order to understand this question, it is necessary that you understand the negative regulation of the *lactose* operon by the *lac* repressor as well as the positive control exerted by the CAP protein. Remember, if lactose is present, it inactivates the *lac* repressor. If glucose is present, it inhibits adenyl cyclase, thereby reducing, through a lowering of cAMP levels, the positive action of CAP on the *lac* operon. **(a)** With no lactose and no glucose, the operon is off because the *lac* repressor is bound to the operator; although CAP is bound to its binding site, it will not override the action of the repressor. **(b)** With lactose added to the medium, the *lac* repressor is inactivated, and the operon is transcribing the structural genes. With no glucose, the CAP is bound to its binding site, thus enhancing transcription. **(c)** With no lactose present in the medium, the *lac* repressor is bound to the operator region, and because glucose inhibits adenyl cyclase, the CAP protein will not interact with its binding site. The operon is therefore "off." **(d)** With lactose present, the *lac* repressor is inactivated; however, because glucose is also present, CAP will not interact with its binding site. Under this condition, transcription is severely diminished and the operon can be considered to be "off."

15-3. Cancer cells often originate under the influence of mutations in tumor suppressor genes or proto-oncogenes. Should hypermetylation occur in one of many DNA repair genes, the frequency of mutation would increase because the DNA repair system is compromised. The resulting increase in mutations might occur in tumor suppressor genes or proto-oncogenes.

15-4. General transcription factors associate with a promoter to stimulate transcription of a specific gene. Some *trans*-acting elements, when bound to enhancers, interact with coactivators to enhance transcription by forming an enhanceosome that stimulates transcription initiation. Transcription can be repressed when certain proteins bind to silencer DNA elements and generate repressive chromatin structures. The same molecule may bind to a different chromosomal regulatory site (enhancer or silencer), depending on the molecular environment of a given tissue type.

Chapter 15 Regulation of Gene Expression

Solutions to Problems and Discussion Questions

1. (a) From 1900 on, scientists have known that when certain additives are supplied to growth media, organisms respond with the production of certain enzymes. Such enzymes were referred to as adaptive in contrast to constitutive enzymes that are produced regardless of particular medium additives.

(b) In most cases, several to many proteins are synthesized or repressed together in response to a given stimulus. Each is often coordinately influenced by a single mutation in a single chromosomal location.

(c) The construction of partial diploid cells, called merozygotes, allowed scientists to determine that regulation can be achieved by agents that are not contiguous with the genes under their control.

(d) Mutations within promoters alter transcription efficiencies whereas deletions alter the initiation point of transcription. Enhancers (and silencers) are chromosomal elements that negatively influence transcription when deleted or altered by mutation. Insertion of an enhancer by recombinant technology increases transcription.

(e) First, for a particular region of a chromosome, there is an inverse relationship between the degree of DNA methylation and the degree of gene expression. Second, DNA methylation patterns are specific for given tissues, thus corresponding with differential gene activity.

2. The answer to this question is key to enhancing a student's understanding of the Jacob-Monod model as related to lactose and tryptophan metabolism. The enzymes of the lactose operon are needed to break down and use lactose as an energy source. If lactose is the sole carbon source, the enzymes are synthesized to use that carbon source. With no lactose present, there is no "need" for the enzymes. The tryptophan operon contains structural genes for the *synthesis* of tryptophan. If there is little or no tryptophan in the medium, the tryptophan operon is "turned on" to manufacture tryptophan. If tryptophan is abundant in the medium, then there is no "need" for the operon to be manufacturing tryptophan synthetases.

3. Refer to F15-1 to see that under *negative* control, the regulatory molecule interferes with transcription, whereas in *positive* control, the regulatory molecule stimulates transcription. Negative control is seen in the *lactose* and *tryptophan* systems. Catabolite repression is an example of positive control. Negative control requires a molecule to be removed from the DNA for transcription to occur. Positive control requires a molecule to be provided to the DNA for transcription to occur.

4. In an *inducible system*, the repressor that normally interacts with the operator to inhibit transcription is inactivated by an *inducer*, thus permitting transcription. In a *repressible system*, a normally inactive repressor is *activated* by a *corepressor*, thus enabling it (the activated repressor) to bind to the operator to inhibit transcription. Because the interaction of the protein (repressor) has a negative influence on transcription, the systems described here are forms of *negative control* (see F15-1).

5. Attenuation involves the formation of exclusive stem-loop structures in the 5'-portion of tryptophan mRNA, where in the presence of excess tryptophan, transcription termination occurs. Attenuation is sensitive to intracellular concentrations of $tRNA^{trp}$. Riboswitches act similarly to attenuation in that a 5' region of a forming mRNA can interact with a ligand (amino acids, metal ions, etc.) to generate a conformation that can form either terminator or antiterminator conformations of transcription.

6. Refer to the text and to F15-1 and F15-2 for a good understanding of the lactose system before starting.

$I^+ O^+ Z^+$ = **inducible** because a repressor protein can interact with the operator to turn off transcription.

$I^- O^+ Z^+$ = **constitutive** because the repressor gene is mutant; therefore, no repressor protein is available.

$I^+ O^c Z^+$ = **constitutive** because even though a repressor protein is made, it cannot bind with the mutant operator.

$I^- O^+ Z^+/F \, 'I^+$ = **inducible** because even though there is one mutant repressor gene, the other I^+ gene, on the F factor, produces a normal repressor protein that is diffusible and capable of interacting with the operon to repress transcription. (See F15-2 in this book.)

$I^+ O^c Z^+/F \, 'O^c$ = **constitutive** because there is a constitutive operator (O^c) next to a normal Z gene. Constitutive synthesis of β-galactosidase will occur.

$I^s O^+ Z^+$ = **repressed** because the product of the I^s gene is *insensitive* to the inducer lactose and thus cannot be inactivated. The repressor will continually interact with the operator and shut off transcription regardless of the presence or absence of lactose.

$I^{s} O^{+} Z^{+}/F\,`I^{+}$ = **repressed** because, as in the previous case, the product of the I^{s} gene is insensitive to the inducer lactose and thus cannot be inactivated. The repressor will continually interact with the operator and shut off transcription regardless of the presence or absence of lactose. The fact that there is a normal I^{+} gene is of no consequence because once a repressor from I^{s} binds to an operator, the presence of normal repressor molecules will make no difference.

7. Refer to the text and to F15-2 for a good understanding of the lactose system before starting.

$I^{+} O^{+} Z^{+}$ = Because of the function of the active repressor from the I^{+} gene, and no lactose to influence its function, there will be **no enzyme made**.

$I^{+} O^{c} Z^{+}$ = There will be a **functional enzyme made** because the constitutive operator is in *cis* with a Z gene. The lactose in the medium will have no influence because of the constitutive operator. The repressor cannot bind to the mutant operator.

$I^{-} O^{+} Z^{-}$ = There will be a **nonfunctional enzyme made** because with I^{-} the system is constitutive, but the Z gene is mutant. The absence of lactose in the medium will have no influence because of the nonfunctional repressor. The mutant repressor cannot bind to the operator.

$I^{-} O^{+} Z^{-}$ = There will be a **nonfunctional enzyme made** because with I^{-} the system is constitutive, but the Z gene is mutant. The lactose in the medium will have no influence because of the nonfunctional repressor. The mutant repressor cannot bind to the operator.

$I^{-} O^{+} Z^{+}/F\,`I^{+}$ = There will be **no enzyme made** because in the absence of lactose, the repressor product of the I^{+} gene will bind to the operator and inhibit transcription.

$I^{+} O^{c} Z^{+}/F\,`O^{+}$ = Because there is a constitutive operator in *cis* with a normal Z gene, there will be **functional enzyme made**. The lactose in the medium will have no influence because of the mutant operator.

$I^{+} O^{+} Z^{-}/F\,`I^{+} O^{+} Z^{+}$ = Because there is lactose in the medium, the repressor protein will not bind to the operator and transcription will occur. The presence of a normal Z gene allows a **functional and nonfunctional enzyme to be made**. The repressor protein is diffusible, working in *trans*.

$I^{-} O^{+} Z^{-}/F\,`I^{+} O^{+} Z^{+}$ = Because there is no lactose in the medium, the repressor protein (from I^{+}) will repress the operators and there will be **no enzyme made**.

$I^{s} O^{+} Z^{+}/F\,`O^{+}$ = With the product of I^{s} there is binding of the repressor to the operator and therefore **no enzyme made**. The lack of lactose in the medium is of no consequence because the mutant repressor is insensitive to lactose.

$I^{+} O^{c} Z^{+}/F\,`O^{+} Z^{+}$ = The arrangement of the constitutive operator (O^{c}) with the Z gene will cause a **functional enzyme to be made**.

8. The mutations described are consistent with the structure of the lac repressor. The N-terminal portion of the repressor is involved in DNA binding, whereas the C-terminal portion is more involved in association with lactose and its analogs.

9. Catabolite repression is a mechanism whereby glucose, a catabolite of lactose, inhibits the synthesis of β-galactosidase. When glucose and lactose are both present, glucose is preferentially used as the energy source. When glucose is exhausted, β-galactosidase synthesis occurs and lactose is metabolized. Thus, catabolite repression balances the use of glucose and lactose through regulation of β-galactosidase synthesis.

10. Generally, cooperative binding occurs when the final outcome is greater than the simple sum of its parts. In the case of transcription factors, each factor has little impact on transcription; however, when all components are present, a cooperative interaction (binding) occurs and a functional complex is made.

11. In order to understand this question, it is necessary that you understand the negative regulation of the *lactose* operon by the *lac* repressor as well as the positive control exerted by the CAP protein. Remember, if lactose is present, it inactivates the *lac* repressor. If glucose is present, it inhibits adenyl cyclase, thereby reducing, through a lowering of cAMP levels, the positive action of CAP on the *lac* operon.

(a) With no lactose and no glucose, the operon is off because the *lac* repressor is bound to the operator, and although CAP is bound to its binding site, it will not override the action of the repressor.

(b) With lactose added to the medium, the *lac* repressor is inactivated and the operon is transcribing

Chapter 15 Regulation of Gene Expression

the structural genes. With no glucose, the CAP is bound to its binding site, thus enhancing transcription.

(c) With no lactose present in the medium, the *lac* repressor is bound to the operator region, and because glucose inhibits adenyl cyclase, the CAP protein will not interact with its binding site. The operon is therefore "off."

(d) With lactose present, the *lac* repressor is inactivated; however, because glucose is also present, CAP will not interact with its binding site. Under this condition, transcription is severely diminished and the operon can be considered to be "off."

12. (a) Because activated CAP is a component of the cooperative binding of RNA polymerase to the *lac* promoter, absence of a functional *crp* would compromise the positive control exhibited by CAP.

(b) Without a CAP binding site, there would be a reduction in the inducibility of the *lac* operon.

13. Attenuation functions to reduce the synthesis of tryptophan when it is in full supply. It does so by reducing transcription of the *tryptophan* operon. The same phenomenon is observed when tryptophan activates the repressor to shut off transcription of the *tryptophan* operon.

14. First, notice that in the first row of data, the presence of tm in the medium causes the production of active enzyme from the wild-type arrangement of genes. From this, one would conclude that the system

is *inducible*. To determine which gene is the structural gene, look for the *IE* function and see that it is related to *C*. Therefore, *C* codes for the **structural gene**. Because when *B* is mutant, no enzyme is produced, *B* must be the **promoter**.

Notice that when genes *A* and *D* are mutant, constitutive synthesis occurs; therefore, one must be the operator and the other gene codes for the repressor protein. To distinguish these functions, one must remember that the repressor operates as a diffusible substance and can be on the host chromosome or the F factor (functioning in *trans*). However, the operator can only operate in *cis*. In addition, in *cis*, the constitutive operator is dominant to its wild-type allele, whereas the mutant repressor is recessive to its wild-type allele.

Notice that the mutant *A* gene is dominant to its wild-type allele, whereas the mutant *d* allele is recessive (behaving as wild type in the first row). Therefore, the *A* locus is the **operator** and the *D* locus is the **repressor** gene.

15. Because the deletion of the regulatory gene causes a loss of synthesis of the enzymes, the regulatory gene product can be viewed as one exerting *positive control*. When tis is present, no enzymes are made; therefore, tis must inactivate the positive regulatory protein. When tis is absent, the regulatory protein is free to exert its positive influence on transcription. Mutations in the operator negate the positive action of the regulator. On the next page is a model that illustrates these points (F15-3).

F15-3 Model of regulatory system described in problem 15. This is an example of *positive* control.

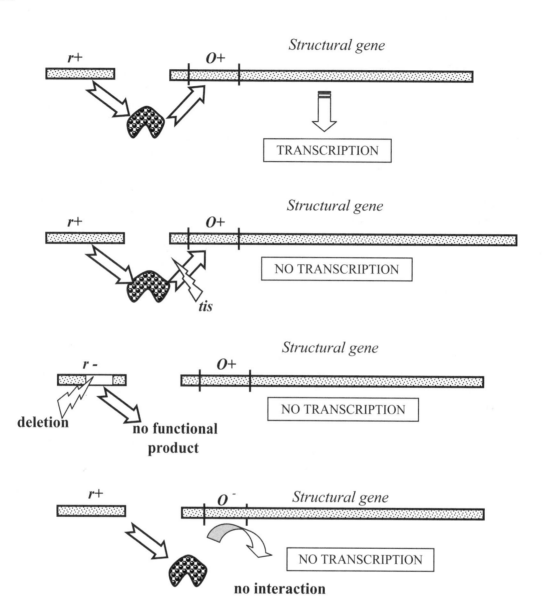

16. The first two sentences of the problem indicate an inducible system in which oil stimulates the production of a protein, which turns on (positive control) genes to metabolize oil. The different results in strains #2 and #4 suggest a *cis*-acting system. Because the operon by itself (when mutant as in strain #3) gives constitutive synthesis of the structural genes, a *cis*-acting system is also supported. The *cis*-acting element is most likely part of the operon.

17. There are several reasons for anticipating a variety of different regulatory mechanisms in eukaryotes as compared with prokaryotes. Eukaryotic cells contain greater amounts of DNA and this DNA is associated with various proteins, including histones and nonhistone chromosomal proteins. *Chromatin* as such does not exist in prokaryotes. In addition, whereas there is usually only one chromosome in prokaryotes, eukaryotes have more than one chromosome all enclosed in a nuclear envelope. This nuclear envelope separates, both temporally and spatially, the processes of transcription and translation, thus providing an opportunity for posttranscriptional, pretranslational regulation.

Whereas prokaryotes respond genetically to changes in their external environment, cells of multicellular eukaryotes interact with each other as well as the external environment. The structural and functional diversity of cells of a multicellular eukaryote, coupled with the finding that all cells of an organism contain a complete complement of genes, suggests that certain genes are active in some cells but not active in other cells.

It is often difficult to study eukaryotic gene regulation because of the complexities mentioned above, especially tissue specificity and the various levels at which regulation can occur (as indicated in questions 20 and 21 below). Obtaining a homogeneous group of cells from a multicellular organism often requires a significant alteration of the natural environment of the cell. Thus, results from studies on isolated cells must be interpreted with caution. In addition, because of the variety of intracellular components (nuclear and cytoplasmic), it is difficult to isolate, free of contamination, certain molecular species. Even if such isolation is accomplished, it is difficult to interpret the actual behavior of such molecules in an artificial environment.

18. *Chromatin remodeling:* Changes in DNA/chromosome structure can influence overall gene output as well as chromosome territories and transcription factories. DNA methylation and histone modifications also influence transcription efficiency.

Transcription: Several factors are known to influence transcription: *promoters*, TATA, CAAT, and GC boxes, as well as other upstream regulatory sequences; *enhancers* and *silencers*, which are *cis*-acting sequences that act at various locations and orientations; *transcription factors*, with various structural motifs that bind DNA and influence transcription; and *receptor-hormone complexes* that influence transcription. Enhancers and silencers are also often involved in regulation. Various transcription factors provide specificity and cooperative interactions with DNA targets.

Processing and transport types of regulation involve the efficiency of pre-mRNA maturation as related to capping, poly-A tail addition, and intron removal. The stability of the mRNAs appears to be an additional regulatory control point. A variety of small molecules are involved in the initiation of transcripton. Certain factors, such as protein subunits, may influence a variety of steps in the translational mechanism. For instance, a protein or protein subunit may activate enzymes that will degrade certain mRNAs, or a particular regulatory element may cause a ribosome to stall, thus decreasing the speed of translation and increasing the exposure of an mRNA to the action of nucleases. Alternative splicing and various forms of RNA interference offer additional points of regulation. Small interfering RNAs and microRNAs may be involved in gene silencing. RNA-directed DNA methylation is also involved in some organisms.

19. *Promoters* are conserved DNA sequences that influence transcription from the "upstream" side (5') of mRNA coding genes. They are usually fixed in position and within 100 base pairs of the initiation site for mRNA synthesis. Examples of such promoter sites are TATA, CAAT, and GC boxes.

Enhancers are *cis*-acting sequences of DNA that stimulate the transcription from most, if not all, promoters. They are somewhat different from promoters in that the position of the enhancer need not be fixed; it may be significantly upstream or downstream or within the gene being regulated. The orientation may be inverted without significantly influencing its action. Enhancers can work on different genes; that is, they are not gene-specific.

20. Transcription factors are proteins that are *necessary* for the initiation of transcription. However, they are not *sufficient* for the initiation of transcription. To be activated, RNA polymerase II requires a number of transcription factors. Transcription factors contain at least two functional domains: one binds to the DNA sequences of promoters and/or enhancers, whereas the other interacts with RNA polymerase or other transcription factors. Some transcription factors bind to other transcription factors without themselves binding to DNA.

21. Your answer should deal with the following issues:

– Differences in basic chromosome structure
– Chromosome remodeling
– Histone acetylation
– Differences in gene structure
– Cell structure (nucleus in eukaryotes)
– Biological context in terms of multicellular
   interactions versus single cell survival

22. Generally, one determines the influence of various regulatory elements by removing necessary elements or adding extra elements. In addition, examining the outcome of mutations within such elements often provides insight as to function. Assay systems determine the relative levels of gene expression after such alterations.

23. RNA interference begins with a double-stranded RNA being processed by a protein called Dicer that, in combination with RISC, generates short interfering RNA (siRNA). Unwinding of siRNA produces an antisense strand that combines with a protein to cleave mRNA complementary sequences. Short RNAs called microRNAs pair with the 3'-untranslated regions of mRNAs and block their translation.

24.

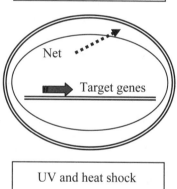

Sketches modified from Ducret et al. *Molecular and Cellular Biology* 1999 19:7076-7087.

25. Methylation of CpGs causes a reduction in luciferase expression, which is somewhat proportional to the amount of methylation and patch size. Methylation within the transcription unit more drastically reduces luciferase expression compared with methylation outside the transcription unit. A high degree of methylation outside the transcription unit (593 CpGs) has as great an impact on depressing transcription as the same degree of methylation within the transcription unit.

26. Following is a sketch of several RNA polymerase molecules (filled circles) in what might be a transcription factory. In this diagram, there are eight RNA pol II molecules shown being transcribed. Nascent transcripts are shown extending from the RNA polymerase molecules. For simplicity, only one promoter is shown and one structural gene is shown.

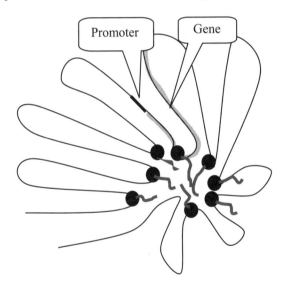

27. When splice specificity is lost, one might observe several classes of altered RNAs: (1) a variety of nonspecific variants producing RNA pools with many lengths and combinations of exons and introns; (2) incomplete splicing whereby introns and exons are erroneously included or excluded in the mRNA product; and (3) a variety of nonsense products, which result in premature RNA decay or truncated protein products. Whether cancer-specific splices initiate or result from tumorigenesis is presently unknown. Given the complexity of cancer induction and the maintenance of the transformed cellular state, gene products that are significant in regulating the cell cycle may certainly be influenced by alternative splicing and thus contribute to cancer.

Chapter 16: The Genetics of Cancer

Concept Areas	Corresponding Problems
Cancer Origins	1, 6, 11, 17, 24, 25, 26
Inherited Cancer	2, 7, 22, 27, 28
Repair Mechanisms	1, 12, 18
Cell-Cycle Dynamics	3, 4, 5, 6
Cancer and the Environment	16, 19, 21
Apoptosis	8
Tumor Suppressors and Oncogenes	9, 10, 13, 14, 18
Chromosome Structure	15, 23
Viruses and Cancer	17, 20

Structures and Processes Checklist – Significant concepts that deserve special attention are identified with a "∗".

(check topic when mastered – provide examples where appropriate – understand the context of each entry)

- **Cancer Is a Genetic Disease**
  - genomic alterations*
  - abnormal cell growth
  - proliferation*
  - metastasis*
  - benign tumor
  - malignant tumor
  - clonal origin*
  - Burkitt's lymphoma
  - X chromosome inactivation
  - cancer stem cell hypothesis*
  - multistep process*
  - multiple mutations*
  - carcinogen*
  - tumorigenesis

- **Genetic Defects/Genomic Stability***
  - mutator phenotype
  - genetic instability
  - chronic myelogenous leukemia*
  - CML
  - Philadelphia chromosome
  - BCR/ABL protein*
  - protein kinase
  - HNPCC*
  - reciprocal translocation*
  - chromatin modifications*
  - cancer epigenetics*
  - histone modifications*

- **Cell-cycle Regulation***
  - apoptosis*
  - signal transduction

- G0 phase
- cell-cycle control
- G1/S checkpoint*
- G2/M checkpoint*
- M checkpoint*
- cyclins*
- cyclin-dependent kinase*
- CDKs*
- programmed cell death*
- **Proto-Oncogenes***
  - tumor-suppressor genes*
  - oncogene*
  - *ras* proto-oncogene
  - *ras* gene family
  - GTP*
  - GDP*
  - *p53*
  - tumor-suppressor gene*
  - cell-cycle arrest
  - *RB1*
  - tumor-suppressor gene*
  - retinoblastoma*
  - retinoblastoma protein
  - pRB*
  - E2F

- **Cancer Cells Metastasize***
  - extracellular matrix
  - basal lamina
  - E-cadherin glycoprotein
  - metalloproteinases*
  - TIMPs*
  - metastasis-suppressor genes
- **Inherited Predisposition***
  - loss of heterozygosity*
  - familial adenomatous polyposis*
  - FAP
  - adenomatous polyposis gene
  - *APC*
  - polyps
  - adenomas
  - transformation
  - *DCC*
- **Viruses Contribute to Cancer***
  - DNA viruses*
  - RNA viruses*
  - retrovirus*
- **Environmental Agents***
  - chemicals
  - radiation
  - tobacco smoke
  - aflatoxin
  - nitrosamines

Answers to Now Solve This

16-1. Several approaches are used to combat CML. One includes the use of a tyrosine kinase inhibitor that binds competitively to the ATP binding site of ABL kinase, thereby inhibiting phosphorylation of BCR/ABL and preventing the activation of additional signaling pathways. In addition, real-time quantitative reverse transcription-polymerase chain reaction (Q-RT-PCR) allows one to monitor drug responses of cell populations in patients so that less toxic and more effective treatments are possible. Being able to distinguish leukemic cells from healthy cells allows one to not only target therapy to specific cell populations, but it also allows for the quantification of responses to therapy. Because such cells produce a hybrid protein, it may be possible to develop a therapy, perhaps an immunotherapy, based on the uniqueness of the BCR/ABL protein.

16-2. *p53* is a tumor suppressor gene that protects cells from multiplying with damaged DNA. It is present in its mutant state in more than 50 percent of all tumors. Because the immediate control of a critical and universal cell cycle checkpoint is mediated by *p53*, mutation will influence a wide range of cell types; *p53*'s action is not limited to specific cell types.

16-3. Cancer is a complex alteration in normal cell-cycle controls. Even if a major "cancer-causing" gene is transmitted, other genes, often new mutations, are usually necessary in order to drive a cell toward tumor formation. Full expression of the cancer phenotype is likely to be the result of interplay among a variety of genes and therefore show variable penetrance and expressivity.

Chapter 16 The Genetics of Cancer

Solutions to Problems and Discussion Questions

1. (a) The clonal origin of cancer cells in a given cancer is supported by findings that mutations, chromosomal or otherwise, are of the same type in all cancerous cells. In addition, the X-chromosome inactivation patterns support the clonal origin of cancer.

(b) The progressive, time- and age-dependent development of tumorigenesis, coupled with the relatively low cancer rate compared to the mutation rate, argues for a multistep mutational model for cancer.

(c) The mutator phenotype, thought by some to be caused by defective DNA repair mechanisms, is characteristic of cancer cells. Numerous cancers, exemplified by xeroderma pigmentosum and hereditary nonpolyposis colorectal cancer, are caused by defective DNA repair systems.

2. Familial retinoblastoma is inherited as an autosomal dominant gene with 90 percent penetrance; that is, 90 percent of the individuals who inherit the gene will develop eye tumors. The gene usually expresses itself in youngsters. Because the husband's sister has RB, one of the husband's parents has the gene for RB and the husband has a 50:50 chance of inheriting that gene. However, because the husband is past the usual age of onset, it is quite likely that he was lucky and did not receive the *RB* gene. In that case, the chance that a child born to this couple having RB is no higher than the frequency of sporadic occurrence. However, because the gene is 90 percent penetrant, there is a chance that the husband has the gene but does not express it. The probability of that occurrence would be 0.50 (chance of inheriting the gene) × 0.10 (not expressing the gene) = 0.05. The chance of the husband then passing this nonexpressed gene to his child would be again 0.50, so 0.50 × 0.05 = 0.025 for the child inheriting this gene. If the child inherits the *RB* gene, he or she has a 90 percent chance of expressing it.

Therefore, the overall probability of the child having RB (using this logic) would be 0.025 × 0.90 = 0.0225, or just over 2 percent (or about 1 in 50).

To test the presence of the *RB* gene in the husband, it is possible in some forms of RB to identify (by molecular probes) a defective or missing DNA segment. Otherwise, one might attempt to assay the RB product in cells to see if it is present and functional at normal levels.

3. Review Chapter 2 in the text and note that the following stages of the cell cycle are discussed: G1, G0, S, and G2. The G1 stage begins after mitosis and is involved in the synthesis of many cytoplasmic elements. In the S phase, DNA synthesis occurs. G2 is a period of growth and preparation for mitosis. Most cell-cycle time variation is caused by changes in the duration of G1. G0 is the nondividing state.

4. The major regulatory points of the cell cycle include the following:

1. late G1 (G1/S)
2. the border between G2 and mitosis (G2/M)
3. mitosis (M)

5. Kinases regulate other proteins by adding phosphate groups. Cyclins bind to the kinases, switching them on and off. CDK4 binds to cyclin D, moving cells from G1 to S. At the G2/mitosis border, a CDK1 (cyclin-dependent kinase) combines with another cyclin (cyclin B). Phosphorylation occurs, bringing about a series of changes in the nuclear membrane via caldesmon, cytoskeleton, and histone H1.

6. The retinoblastoma gene (*RB1*), located on chromosome 13, encodes a protein designated pRB. Cells progress through the G1/S transition when pRB is phosphorylated and CDK4 binds to cyclin D. In the absence of phosphorylation of pRB, it binds to members of the E2F family of transcription factors, which controls the expression of genes required to move the cell from G1 to S. When E2F and other regulators are released by pRB, they are free to induce the expression of more than 30 genes whose products are required for the transition from G1 into S phase. After cells traverse S, G2, and M phases, pRB reverts to a nonphosphorylated state, binds to regulatory proteins such as E2F, and keeps them sequestered until required for the next cell cycle.

7. To say that a particular trait is inherited conveys the assumption that when a particular genetic circumstance is present, it will be revealed in the phenotype. For instance, albinism is inherited in such a way that individuals who are homozygous recessive express albinism. When one discusses an inherited predisposition, one usually refers to situations in which a particular phenotype is expressed in families in some consistent pattern. However, the phenotype may not always be expressed or may manifest itself in different ways. In retinoblastoma, the gene is inherited as an autosomal dominant, and those who inherit the mutant *RB* allele are predisposed to develop eye tumors. However, approximately 10 percent of the people known to inherit the gene do not actually express it, and in some cases expression involves only one eye, rather than two.

8. Apoptosis, or programmed cell death, is a genetically controlled process that leads to death of a cell. It is a natural process involved in morphogenesis and a protective mechanism against cancer formation. During apoptosis, nuclear DNA becomes fragmented, cellular structures are disrupted, and the cells are dissolved. Caspases are involved in the initiation and progress of apoptosis.

9. A tumor-suppressor gene is a gene that normally functions to suppress cell division. Because tumors and cancers represent a significant threat to survival and therefore Darwinian fitness, strong evolutionary forces would favor a variety of co-evolved and perhaps complex conditions in which mutations in these suppressor genes would be recessive. Looking at it in another way, if a tumor-suppressor gene makes a product that regulates the cell cycle favorably, cellular conditions have evolved in such a way that sufficient quantities of this gene product are made from just one allele (of the two present in each diploid individual) to provide normal function.

10. The nonphosphorylated form of pRB binds to transcription factors such as E2F, causing inactivation and suppression of the cell cycle. Phosphorylation of pRB activates the cell cycle by releasing transcription factors (E2F) to advance the cell cycle. With the phosphorylation site inactivated in the PSM-RB form, phosphorylation cannot occur, thereby leaving the cell cycle in a suppressed state.

11. Imbedded in the plasma membrane, Ras proteins act as molecular switches that transmit molecular signals from outside to inside the cell. Activated Ras proteins tranduce a signal, which activates the transcription of genes that start cell division. Mutant Ras proteins are locked into the "on" position, continually signaling cell division.

12. Various kinases can be activated by breaks in DNA. One kinase, called ATM, and/or a kinase called Chk2 phosphorylates BRCA1 and p53. The activated p53 arrests replication during the S phase to facilitate DNA repair. The activated BRCA1 protein, in conjunction with BRCA2, mRAD51, and other nuclear proteins, is involved in repairing the DNA.

13. Oncogenes are genes that induce or maintain uncontrolled cellular proliferation associated with cancer. They are mutant forms of proto-oncogenes, which normally function to regulate cell division. Oncogenes may be formed through point mutations, gene amplification, translocations, repositioning of regulatory sequences, or other mechanisms.

14. Mutations that produce oncogenes alter gene expression either directly or indirectly and act in a dominant capacity. Proto-oncogenes are those that normally function to promote or maintain cell division. In the mutant state (oncogenes), they induce or maintain uncontrolled cell division; that is, there is a gain of function. Generally, this gain of function takes the form of increased or abnormally continuous gene output. On the other hand, loss of function is generally attributed to mutations in tumor-suppressor genes, which function to halt passage through the cell cycle. When such genes are mutant, they have lost their capacity to halt the cell cycle. Such mutations are generally recessive.

15. A translocation involving exchange of genetic material between chromosomes 9 and 22 is responsible for the generation of the "Philadelphia chromosome." Genetic mapping established that certain genes were combined to form a hybrid oncogene (*BCR/ABL*) that encodes a 200-kDa protein that has been implicated in the formation of chronic myelogenous leukemia.

16. Unfortunately, it is common to spend enormous amounts of money dealing with diseases after they occur rather than concentrating on disease prevention. Too often, pressure from special interest groups or lack of political stimulus retards advances in education and prevention. Obviously, it is less expensive, in terms of both human suffering and money, to seek preventive measures for as many diseases as possible. However, having gained some understanding of the mechanisms of disease, in this case cancer, it must also be stated that no matter what preventive measures are taken, it will be impossible to completely eliminate disease from the human population. It is extremely important, however, that we increase efforts to educate and protect the human population from as many hazardous environmental agents as possible.

17. Because the evolutionary strategy of a virus is to promote its own replication, and because it does so in a host cell, stimulating cell division in host cells confers an evolutionary advantage. To encourage infected cells to undergo growth and division, viruses often encode genes that stimulate growth and division. Many viruses either inactivate tumor suppressor genes of the host or bring in genes that stimulate cell growth and division. By inactivating tumor suppressor genes, the normal breaking mechanism of the cell cycle is destroyed.

18. Normal cells are often capable of withstanding mutational assault because they have checkpoints and DNA repair mechanisms in place. When such mechanisms fail, cancer may be a result. Through mutation, such protective mechanisms are compromised in cancer cells, and as a result, they show higher than normal rates of mutation, chromosomal abnormalities, and genomic instability.

19. An acute transforming virus is a retrovirus that carries an oncogene(s), whereas a nonacute virus can induce the activity of cellular genes that bring about tumor formation.

20. Certain environmental agents such as chemicals and X rays cause mutations. Because genes control the cell cycle, mutations in cell-cycle control genes, or those that impact cell-cycle control, can lead to cancer.

21. Radiotherapy is often administered externally or internally to damage the cell-cycle machinery, thus shrinking the cancer or killing cells of the cancer. It may be completely or partially effective. Because cells have natural defenses against mutagenic insult, drugs that increase a cell's sensitivity to radiation may be administered. Radiosensitizers and radioprotectors are chemicals that alter a cell's response to radiotherapy. Radiosensitizers make cells more sensitive to therapy, whereas radioprotectors are drugs that protect normal cells from the damage caused by radiation therapy. Radiotherapy kills cells; therefore, side effects are expected.

22. No, she will still have the general population risk of about 10 percent. In addition, it is possible that genetic tests will not detect all breast cancer mutations.

23. Because there are multiple routes that lead to cancer, one would expect complex regulatory systems to be involved. More specifically, whereas in some cases, down regulation of a gene, such as an oncogene, may be a reasonable cancer therapy, down regulation of a tumor suppressor gene would be undesirable in therapy. Various levels of methylation (hypermethylation and hypomethylation) influence gene activity and therefore can cause cancer.

24. A benign tumor is a multicellular cell mass that is usually localized to a given anatomical site. Malignant tumors are those generated by cells that have migrated to one or more secondary sites. Malignant tumors are more difficult to treat and can be life-threatening.

25. Proteases in general and serine proteases specifically are considered tumor-promoting agents because they degrade proteins, especially those in the extracellular matrix. When such proteolysis occurs, cellular invasion and metastasis are encouraged. Consistent with this observation are numerous observations that metastatic tumor cells are associated with higher than normal amounts of protease expression. Inhibitors of serine proteases are often tested for their anticancer efficacy.

26. As with many forms of cancer, a single gene alteration is not the only requirement. The authors (Bose et al.) state "but only infrequently do the cells acquire the additional changes necessary to produce leukemia in humans." Some studies indicate that variations (often deletions) in the region of the breakpoints may influence expression of CML.

27. **(a)** Because one is working with somatic cells, the usual tests for heterozygosity through crosses are not available. Therefore, one must rely on chemical/physical approaches to answer the question. A genomic library could be constructed of both osteosarcoma cell DNA and noncancerous cells from the same organism. You could then screen the library using labeled probes from the clones carrying the *RB1* gene available to you as stated in the problem. At this point, some indications might emerge because if there is a significant alteration in mutant *RB1* genes, probes may not successfully hybridize to any clones in the cancerous cell DNA library. Assuming that control hybridization occurs in the noncancerous cells, lack of hybridization in the library derived from the osteosarcoma cell line might indicate deletions. However, assuming that hybridization does allow one to identify clones containing putative *RB1* alleles, subcloning into appropriate vectors would allow sequencing to reveal sequence changes in the *RB1* alleles when compared with nonmutant genes.

A second approach combines an immunoassay described in part (b) of this problem. Assuming that one can successfully make antibodies to the normal *RB1* gene product (pRB), lack of cross-reactivity of the pRB antibodies to proteins from the cancerous cell line would indicate that both *RB1* alleles are mutant.

(b) As indicated in the last portion of part (a) above, one can make antibodies to pRB from the noncancerous cells and test these antibodies for reactivity against proteins from the cancerous cell lines. A pRB-antibody reaction would indicate that the pRB protein is made.

(c) To determine whether addition of a normal *RB1* gene will change the cancer-causing potential of osteosarcoma cells, one could transfer the cloned normal *RB1* gene into the cells by transformation or transfection (often by electroporation or ultrasound).

Transformed cells would then be introduced into the cancer-prone mice to determine whether their cancer-causing potential had been altered.

28. (a, b) Even though there are changes in the *BRCA1* gene, they do not always have physiological consequences. Such neutral polymorphisms make screening difficult in that one cannot always be certain that a mutation will cause problems for the patient.

(c) The polymorphism in *PM2* is probably a silent mutation because the third base of the codon is involved.

(d) The polymorphism in *PM3* is probably a neutral missense mutation because the first base is involved. However, because there is some first codon position degeneracy, it is possible for the mutation to be silent.

Chapter 17: Recombinant DNA Technology

Concept Areas	Corresponding Problems
Overview	8
Making DNA Clones	1, 3, 4, 7, 11
Restriction Endonucleases	1, 2, 5, 6
Constructing DNA Libraries	1, 13, 15
Identifying Specific Cloned Sequences	9, 12, 19
DNA Sequencing	18
Polymerase Chain Reaction	1, 10, 16, 17, 21
Applications	14, 19, 20, 22

Structures and Processes Checklist – Significant concepts that deserve special attention are identified with a "∗".

(check topic when mastered – provide examples where appropriate – understand the context of each entry)

- **Recombinant DNA**
  - clone*
- **Recombinant DNA Technology**
  - restriction enzyme*
  - DNA cloning vector*
  - recognition sequence*
  - restriction site*
  - palindrome*
  - cohesive ends
  - blunt end
  - anneal
  - DNA ligase
  - cloning vector
  - selectable marker gene*
  - plasmid vector
  - transformation*

- electroporation
- multiple cloning site*
- phosphodiester bond
- DNA nicks
- blue-white selection*
- *lacZ* gene*
- β-galactosidase*
- λ phage
- bacterial artificial chromosome
- BAC
- yeast artificial chromosome
- YAC
- expression vector
- Ti plasmid
- **DNA Libraries***
  - genomic library*

Chapter 17 Recombinant DNA Technology

- whole-genome shotgun cloning*
- cDNA libraries*
- complementary DNA
- reverse transcriptase*
- screening the library*
- probe*
- hybridization*
- **Polymerase Chain Reaction***
  - PCR
  - primers
  - target DNA
  - cycle*
  - denaturation*
  - hybridization/annealing*
  - extension
  - thermocyclers
  - *Taq* polymerase*
  - limitations of PCR*
  - applications of PCR*
  - reverse transcription PCR

- RT-PCR
- quantitative real-time PCR
- qPCR
- **Analyzing DNA***
  - restriction mapping*
  - nucleic acid blotting*
  - Southern blot*
  - Northern blot
  - Western blot
  - fluorescent in situ hybridization*
  - FISH
- **DNA Sequencing***
  - dideoxynucleotide chain-termination
  - Sanger sequencing
  - dideoxynucleotide*
  - ddNTP*
  - high-throughput DNA sequencing
  - next-generation sequencing
  - NGS
  - SOLiD

Answers to Now Solve This

17-1. (a) Because the *Drosophila* DNA has been cloned into the *Pst*I site in the ampicillin resistance gene of the plasmid, the gene will be mutated and any bacterium with the recombinant plasmid will be ampicillin sensitive. The tetracycline resistance gene remains active, however. Bacteria that have been transformed with the recombinant plasmid will be resistant to tetracycline and therefore tetracycline should be added to the medium.

(b) Colonies that grow on a tetracycline medium only should contain the insert. Those bacteria that do not grow on the ampicillin medium probably contain the *Drosophila* DNA insert.

(c) Resistance to both antibiotics by a transformed bacterium could be explained in several ways. First, if cleavage with the *Pst*I was incomplete, then no change in biological properties of the uncut plasmids would be expected. Also, it is possible that the cut ends of the plasmid were ligated together in the original form with no insert.

17-2. Because the African okapi is a mammal (relative of the giraffe), it will have many sequences in common with those of humans and other mammals that have been sequenced. Using the human nucleotide sequence, for example, one can produce primers that are likely to be useful for isolating particular genes. If primers identical to humans are not successful, then a series of degenerate primers might be used.

Chapter 17 Recombinant DNA Technology

Solutions to Problems and Discussion Questions

1. (a) In general, when DNA fragments of interest have been incorporated into a plasmid, the result is a change in the function of a gene or genes in the plasmid. For instance, if one inserts a piece of DNA into the ampicillin resistance gene, following transformation, the bacterium is no longer resistant to ampicillin. Other techniques involving "insertional mutagenesis" might involve using a medium-driven color change in bacteria that contain a recombinant plasmid.

(b) The choice of method often depends on a variety of circumstances. Sometimes probes are used to screen a library. Such probes may be used to identify particular genes in gels or from membranes containing DNA from lysed bacteria. If appropriate primers are available, PCR can be used to identify particular genes of interest.

(c) Purified genomic DNA is first denatured, and then annealed to specific primers. Once primers have annealed, they are extended. The process is repeated to give many copies of a specific DNA molecule.

(d) Whereas earlier advances relied on single-tube, fluorescent labeling technologies, newer approaches involved solid-phase methodologies in which beads are attached to DNA fragments and amplified by PCR in water droplets in oil. Next-generation sequencing technologies (NGS) have greatly accelerated sequencing, whereas new trends often involve nanotechnology and solid support systems. The overall goal is to increase the speed and accuracy of sequencing while reducing the per base cost.

2. Recombinant DNA technology, also called genetic engineering or gene splicing, involves the creation of associations of DNA that are not typically found in nature. Particular enzymes called *restriction endonucleases* cut DNA at specific sites and often yield "sticky" ends for additional interaction with DNA molecules cut with the same class of enzyme.

  Isolated from bacteria, restriction enzymes fall into several classes, each having peculiarities as to structure and interaction with DNA. A vector may be a plasmid, bacteriophage, or cosmid that receives, through ligation, a piece or pieces of foreign DNA. The recombinant vector can transform (or transfect) a host cell (bacterium, yeast cell, etc.) and be amplified in number.

3. In a DNA cloning experiment, DNA ligase is used to generate the covalent bonds of the phosphodiester backbone to yield an intact double-stranded DNA molecule. Restriction enzymes, on the other hand, break such bonds.

4. Although bacteria are commonly used in cloning, other cell types are also very useful, such as yeast, mammalian, and so on. Bacteria are prokaryotes and as such do not process transcripts as do eukaryotes; therefore, there is often an advantage to using a eukaryotic host. In addition, one might be interested in the influence of a specific DNA segment in a specific host environment, thus necessitating the use of a variety of hosts.

5. This segment contains the palindromic sequence of GGATCC, which is recognized by the restriction enzyme *Bam*HI. The double-stranded sequence is the following:

5'GGATCC
3'CCTAGG

6. The simple answer to this question is to assume that one is asking about the advantage to the scientist of having restriction enzyme sites recognize palindromic sites. In this case, the answer would be that single-stranded overhanging ends are often generated, which allow DNA from different sources cut with the same restriction enzyme to generate complementary overhangs, which can anneal to form recombinant molecules.

  If one considers the question from a bacterial standpoint, the answer is much more involved. In fact, bacterial chromosomes actually have fewer palindromic sites than expected based on chance. This adaptation stems from the fact that restriction sites cleave at palindromic sequences, and one way to keep them from cleaving the host DNA is to evolve away from such sequences. So why do restriction enzymes often cleave at palindromic sites in the first place? First, the classical Type II restriction enzymes are dimers of identical units that recognize identical sequences. To protect such sequences in the bacterial chromosome from attack, a modification enzyme, a methyltransferase, must fully methylate certain bases on both strands of the DNA at the site of a particular restriction endonuclease attack.

Methyltransferases are typically monomers consistent with the process of methylating newly replicated DNA strands. In order for both strands to be protected by methylation, the sequence must be read the same in both directions on the double helix. So, returning to the original question, the advantage to the bacterium of having palindromic sites for restriction enzymes is related more to the protection of such sites from cleavage.

7. Plasmids were the first to be used as cloning vectors, and they are still routinely used to clone relatively small fragments of DNA. Because of their small size, they are relatively easy to separate from the host bacterial chromosome, and they have relatively few restriction sites. They can be engineered fairly easily (*i.e.,* polylinkers and reporter genes added). For cloning larger pieces of DNA such as entire eukaryotic genes, cosmids are often used. For instance, when modifications are made in the bacterial virus lambda (λ), relatively large inserts of about 20kb can be cloned. This is an important advantage when one needs to clone a large gene or generate a genomic library from a eukaryote.

8. No. The tumor-inducing plasmid (Ti) that is used to produce genetically modified plants is specific for the bacterium *Agrobacterium tumifaciens,* which causes tumors in many plant species. There is no danger that this tumor-inducing plasmid will cause tumors in humans.

9. A probe is any DNA or RNA that is complementary to some part of a target gene or sequence. Probes are used to identify and/or locate a particular nucleic acid sequence among a pool of sequences.

10. The total number of molecules after 15 cycles would be 16,384 or $(2)^{14}$.

11. Given that there is only one site for the action of *Hind*III, the following will occur: Cuts will be made such that a four-base single-stranded set of sticky ends will be produced. For the antibiotic resistance to be present, the ligation will reform the plasmid into its original form. However, two of the plasmids can join to form a dimer as indicated in the following diagram.

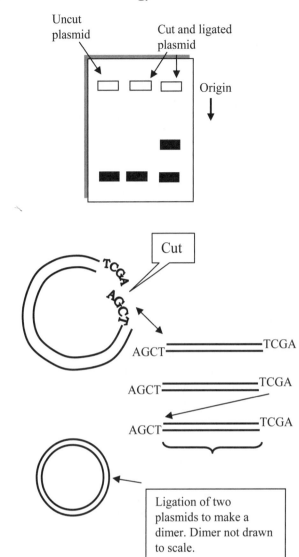

Ligation of two plasmids to make a dimer. Dimer not drawn to scale.

12. Using the human nucleotide sequence, one can produce a probe to screen the library of the African okapi. Second, one can use the amino acid sequence and the genetic code to generate a complementary DNA probe for screening of the library. The probe is used, through hybridization, to identify the DNA that is complementary to the probe and to allow one to identify the library clone containing the DNA of interest. Cells with the desired clone are then picked from the original plate, and the plasmid is isolated from the cells.

13. A cDNA library provides DNAs from RNA transcripts and is therefore useful in identifying what are likely to be functional DNA. If one desires an examination of non-coding as well as coding regions, a genomic library would be more useful.

14. Option (b) fits the expectation because the thick band in the offspring probably represents the bands at approximately the same position in both parents. The likelihood of such a match is expected to be low in the general population.

15. Assuming that one has knowledge of the amino acid sequence of the protein product or the nucleotide sequence of the target nucleic acid, a degenerate set of DNA strands can be made that can be prepared for cloning into an appropriate vector or amplified by PCR. A variety of labeling techniques can then be used, through hybridization, to identify complementary base sequences contained in the genomic library. One must know at least a portion of the amino acid sequence of the protein product or its nucleic acid sequence in order for the procedure to be applied. Some problems can occur through degeneracy in the genetic code (not allowing construction of an appropriate probe), the possible existence of pseudogenes in the library (hybridizations with inappropriate related fragments in the library), and variability of DNA sequences in the library due to introns (causing poor or background hybridization). To overcome some of these problems, one can construct a variety of relatively small probes of different types that take into account the degeneracy in the code. By varying the conditions of hybridization (salt and temperature) one can reduce undesired hybridizations.

16. (a) Heating to 90–95^{0}C denatures the double-stranded DNA so that it dissociates into single strands. It usually takes about five minutes, depending on the length and GC content of the DNA.

(b) Lowering the temperature to 50–70^{0}C allows the primers to bind to the denatured DNA.

(c) Bringing the temperature to 70–75^{0}C allows the heat-stable DNA polymerase an opportunity to extend the primers by adding nucleotides to the 3' ends of each growing strand. Each PCR is designed with specific temperatures (not ranges) based on the characteristics of the DNAs (template and primers).

17. *Taq* polymerase is from a bacterium called *Thermus aquaticus*, which typically lives in hot springs. It is heat stable like some other enzymes used in PCR that are isolated from thermal vents in the ocean floor.

18. ddNTPs are analogs of the "normal" deoxyribonucleotide triphosphates (dNTPs), but they lack a 3'-hydroxyl group. As DNA synthesis occurs, the DNA polymerase occasionally inserts a ddNTP into a growing DNA strand. Because there is no 3'-hydroxyl group, chain elongation cannot take place and resulting fragments are formed, which can be separated by electrophoresis. Where the ddNTP was incorporated, the length of each strand, and therefore the position of the particular ddNTP, is established and used to eventually provide the base sequence of the DNA.

19. FISH involves the hybridization of a labeled probe to a complementary stretch of DNA in a chromosome. As such, it can be used to locate a specific DNA sequence (often a gene or gene fragment) in a chromosome. Spectral karyotyping uses FISH to detect individual chromosomes, a distinct advantage in identifying chromosomal abnormalities.

20. (a) The overall size of the fragment is 12kb. From the A + N digest, sites A and N must be 1kb apart. N must be 2kb from an E site. Pattern #5 is the likely choice. Notice that digest A + N breaks up the 6kb E fragment.

(b) By drawing lines though sections that hybridize to the probe, one can see that the only place of consistent overlap to the probe is the 1kb fragment between A and N.

21. $T_m(^oC) = 81.5 + 0.41(\%GC) - (675/N) = 81.5 + 0.41(33.3) - (675/21) = $ about 63^{0}C. Subtracting 5^{0}C gives us a good starting point of about 58^{0}C for PCR with this primer. Notice that as the percentage of GC and length increase, the $T_m(^oC)$ increases. GC pairs contain three hydrogen bonds rather than two as between AT pairs.

22. (a) Short tandem repeats of the Y chromosome (Y-STRs) vary considerably among individuals and populations. By amplifying Y-STRs by PCR and separating the amplified products by electrophoresis, one can genotypically type an individual as one does with a standard fingerprint. Because tissue samples are often left at the scene of a violent crime, DNA fingerprints are sometimes more available than standard fingerprints. Linking an individual with the time and place of a significant event has multiple forensic applications. Eliminating an individual as a suspect also has important forensic applications.

(b) The nonrecombining region of the Y is maintained strictly in the male population. Of special relevance in forensic applications would be the elimination of half the population (females) from a suspect group.

(c) Because different ethnic groups show different levels of Y-STR polymorphism, different final probabilities occur as products of individual probabilities. Because these probabilities are used to match individuals in forensics, ethnic variations must be taken under consideration.

(d) Although there are many potential uses of DNA samples, generally a "match" is determined by multiplying the occurrence probabilites of each haplotype to arrive at the overall probability (product) of a genotype occurring in a population. If an individual's genotype matches that found in DNA at a crime scene, depending on the frequencies of the haplotypes, one might be able to say that the individual was at the crime scene. However, contamination, inappropriate genotyping, and laboratory expertise may give both false positive or negative results. Identical twins will have identical DNA fingerprints and may complicate forensic applications.

Chapter 18: Genomics, Bioinformatics, and Proteomics

Concept Areas	Corresponding Problems
Genomics Overview	1, 3, 19, 21
Human Genome Project	5, 8, 9, 10, 12, 13
Sequencing	1, 6, 18
Genomic Organization	1, 19, 20, 22
Bioinformatics	1, 2, 4, 7, 20, 21, 22
Proteomics	14, 15
Annotation	1, 11, 17
Microarrays	1, 16

Structures and Processes Checklist – Significant concepts that deserve special attention are identified with a "*".

(check topic when mastered – provide examples where appropriate – understand the context of each entry)

- **Genome**
  - genomics*
- **Whole-Genome Shotgun Sequencing***
  - structural genomics*
  - partial digests
  - contiguous fragments*
  - contig
  - alignment*
  - The Institute for Genome Research
  - TIGR
  - computer-automated sequencing
  - high-throughput sequencing
- **Analysis Relies on Bioinformatics***
  - bioinformatics*
  - domains
  - motifs

- GenBank
- NIH
- NCBI
- accession number
- annotation*
- BLAST*
- similarity score*
- identity value
- hallmark characteristics of a gene*
- exons
- introns
- TATA box
- GC box
- open reading frame
- ORF
- initiation sequence
- termination sequence

- **Functional Genomics***
  - predicting function*
  - homologous genes*
  - orthologs*
  - paralogs*
  - protein domains*
  - motifs
  - Human Genome Project
  - *CFTR* gene
  - ELSI program
  - Celera Genomics
  - features of the human genome*
  - approximately 20,000 genes*
  - approximately 100,000 proteins*
  - alternative splicing*
  - SNPs*
  - CNVs*
- **Omics Revolution***
  - proteomics
  - metabolomics
  - glycomics
  - toxicogenomics
  - metagenomics
  - pharmacogenomics
  - transcriptomics
  - nutrigenomics
  - stone-age genomics
  - ENCODE project
  - personalized genomics
- PGP*
- human microbiome project*
- genome 10K plan*
- **Comparative Genomics***
  - prokaryotic and eukaryotic genomes*
  - gene density*
  - introns*
  - repetitive sequences*
  - model organisms*
  - dog genome*
  - chimpanzee genome*
  - Rhesus monkey genome*
  - sea urchin genome*
  - pseudogenes*
  - Neanderthal genome*
  - evolution*
  - multigene families*
  - superfamily*
  - globin gene*
  - myoglobin gene*
  - hemoglobin*
  - β-globin*
- **Metagenomics***
  - environmental genomics*
  - GOS expedition
- **Transcriptome Analysis***
  - transcriptomics
  - global analysis of gene expression*
  - DNA microarray analysis*

- gene chips
- ESTs*
- cDNA*
- sea urchin development*
- **Proteomics of Cells***
  - proteome*
  - proteomics
  - clinical interest
  - human proteome*
  - 150,000–200,000 proteins
  - dynamic changes*
  - processing
- **Protein Structure Initiative***
  - PSI
  - technologies
- 2DGE*
- isoelectric focusing*
- SDS-PAGE*
- 2D gel*
- mass spectrometry*
- mass-to-charge ratio
- m/z
- MALDI
- protein microarrays
- collagen in *T. rex*
- **Systems Biology***
  - integrated approach
  - interactome
  - network map*

Answers to Now Solve This

18-1. (a,b) Most eukaryotic genes are organized in a particular manner and contain coding segments (exons), noncoding segments (introns), enhancers, promoters, untranslated regions (UTRs), and gene termination sequences. Protein-coding genes often contain one or more open-reading frames that are translated into an amino acid sequence of a protein. Such regions typically begin with a ATG (start codon) and end in some termination sequence (stop codons). It is through these types of landmarks that genes are typically identified. **(b)** Eight percent of 20,000 is 1600. Therefore, one would concluded that chromosome 1 is gene rich.

18-2. Because structural and chemical factors determine the function of a protein, it is likely to have several proteins share a considerable amino acid sequence identity, but not be functionally identical. Because the *in vivo* function of such a protein is determined by secondary and tertiary structures, as well as local surface chemistries in active or functional sites, the non-identical sequences may have considerable influence on function. Note that the query matches to different site positions within the target proteins. A number of other factors suggesting different functions include associations with other molecules (cytoplasmic, membrane, or extracellular), chemical nature and position of binding domains, posttranslational modification, signal sequences, and so on.

18-3. Because blood is relatively easy to obtain in a pure state, its components can be analyzed without fear of tissue-site contamination. Second, blood is intimately exposed to virtually all cells of the body and may therefore carry chemical markers to certain abnormal cells it represents, theoretically, an ideal probe into the human body. However, when blood is removed from the body, its proteome changes and those changes are dependent on a number of environmental factors. Thus, what might be a valid diagnostic for one condition might not be so under others. In addition, the serum proteome is subject to change depending on the genetic, physiologic, and environmental state of the patient. Age and sex are additional variables that must be considered. Validation of a plasma proteome for a particular cancer would be strengthened by demonstrating that the stage of development of the cancer correlates with a commensurate change in the proteome in a relatively large, statistically significant pool of patients. Second, the types of changes in the proteome should be reproducible and, at least until complexities are clarified, involve tumorigenic proteins. It would be helpful to have comparisons with archived samples of each individual at a disease-free time.

Chapter 18 Genomics, Bioinformatics, and Proteomics
Solutions to Problems and Discussion Questions

1. (a) Generally, contigs are suspected to be part of the same chromosome in that their end sequences overlap.

(b) Identification of a protein-coding region is suspected if similar sequences are conserved in other species and various upstream, downstream, splicing, and punctuation sequences are present and appropriately in the proper reading frames.

(c) Comparisons of base sequence data with other organisms indicate conservation of a considerable number of sequences. Because of such conservation, functional relationships are strongly supported. Adding additional support are comparative mutation analyses indicating similar function.

(d) Proteomics is the identification and analysis of proteins in cells, tissues, and organisms. Genome annotation provides an estimate of the number of protein coding genes, whereas a number of sophisticated techniques including electrophoresis, chromatography, spectrophotometry, and microarrays indicate the number of proteins actually produced. The finding that there are many more types of proteins than genes in the genome has generated a number of explanations.

(e) By comparing the amino acid sequences of proteins, the base sequences of genes, and intron/exon architecture, researchers have determined that many genes originated by duplication. Sequence divergence often alters duplicated genes, thus providing the raw material for the evolution of new genes.

(f) Microarrays provide a method for identifying active genes by the hybridization of complementary gene products to stretches of DNA. Different hybridization patterns indicate that whereas some genes are expressed in almost all cells, others show cell- and tissue-specific expression.

2. Functional genomics seeks to understand functional components with the genome and similarities of genomes across phylogenetic and evolutionary distances. Comparative genomics analyzes the arrangement and organization of families of genes within and among genomes.

3. Genomes of both types of organisms are composed of double-stranded DNA (larger in eukaryotes) associated with proteins (more transient in prokaryotes). Both contain open reading frames, but those of prokaryotes are more densely packed. Both have some genes in clusters, but they are much more pronounced in prokaryotes (operons). There are a few repetitive sequences in prokaryotes, but this trend is much more common in eukaryotes. Both contain informational sequences, but those of eukaryotes are often interrupted (introns). Almost all genomes contain transposable elements.

4. Understanding the genome is dependent on the field of bioinformatics, in which computer and mathematics applications are used to organize, share, and analyze data generated by sequencing data. World access to such data is dependent on the ability to store, efficiently share, and obtain the maximum amount of information from protein and DNA sequences. As genomics emerged, bioinformatics became a significant player and today occupies an intellectual enterprise that fuses biological data with information technology, mathematics, and statistical analysis. Most applications, such as the identification of informational content in the genome and DNA sequencing, rely on sequence alignments in nucleic acids and proteins.

5. The main goals of the Human Genome Project are to establish, categorize, and analyze functions for human genes:

- To establish functional categories for all human genes

- To analyze genetic variations between humans, including the identification of single-nucleotide polymorphisms (SNPs)

- To map and sequence the genomes of several model organisms used in experimental genetics, including *E. coli*, *S. cerevisiae*, *C. elegans*, *D. melanogaster*, and *M. musculus* (the mouse)

- To develop new sequencing technologies, such as high-throughput computer-automated sequencers, to facilitate genome analysis

- To disseminate genome information, both among scientists and to the general public

Two of the biggest surprises regarding the HGP were that only a relatively small percentage of the human genome codes for proteins and at least half of the genes show sequence similarity to genes of other organisms.

6. High-throughput technologies allow comprehensive analyses of a number of labor-intensive tasks that would normally take days or weeks to be reduced to half-day activities. By shortening sequencing times for examples, numerous organisms can be sequenced to yield highly informative comparative sequences (comparative genomics). Applied to both genomics and proteomics, high-throughput technologies allow rapid analyses and deployment of genomic information.

7. One initial approach to annotating a sequence is to compare the newly sequenced genomic DNA to the known sequences already stored in various databases. The National Center for Biotechnology Information (NCBI) provides access to BLAST (Basic Local Alignment Search Tool) software that directs searches through databanks of DNA and protein sequences. A segment of DNA can be compared to sequences in major databases such as GenBank to identify matches that align in whole or in part. One might seek similarities of a sequence on chromosome 11 in a mouse and find that or similar sequences in a number of taxa. BLAST will compute a similarity score or identity value to indicate the degree to which two sequences are similar. BLAST is one of many sequence alignment algorithms (RNA-RNA, protein-protein, etc.) that may sacrifice sensitivity for speed.

8. The human genome is composed of more than 3 billion nucleotides in which about 2 percent code for genes. Genes are unevenly distributed over chromosomes with gene-rich clusters separated by gene-poor ones (deserts). Human genes tend to be larger and contain more and larger introns than those in invertebrates such as *Drosophila*. It is estimated that at least half of the genes generate products by alternative splicing. Hundreds of genes have been transferred from bacteria into vertebrates. Duplicated regions are common, which may facilitate chromosomal rearrangement. The human genome appears to contain approximately 20,000 protein-coding genes; however, there is still uncertainty as to the total number.

9. Bacterial genes are densely packed in the chromosome. The protein-coding genes are mostly organized in polycistronic transcription units without introns. Eukaryotic genes are less densely packed in chromosomes, and protein-coding genes are mostly organized as single transcription units with introns.

10. Because many repetitive regions of the genome are not directly involved in production of a phenotype, they tend to be isolated from selection and show considerable variation in redundancy. Length variation in such repeats is unique among individuals (except for identical twins) and, with various detection methods, provides the basis for DNA fingerprinting. Single nucleotide polymorphisms also occur frequently in the genome and can be used to distinguish individuals.

11. One usually begins to annotate a sequence by comparing it, often using BLAST, to the known sequences already stored in various databases. Similarity to other annotated sequences often provides insight as to a sequences function. Hallmarks to annotation are the identification of gene regulatory sequences found upstream of genes (promoters, enhancers, and silencers) downstream elements (termination sequences) and triplet nucleotides that are part of the coding region of the gene. In addition, 5' and 3' splice sites that are used to distinguish exons from introns as well as polyadenylation sites are also used in annotation. Similar hallmarks are used to annotate procaryotic genes; however, because prokaryotic genes don't contain introns, their annotation is sometimes less complicated. Annotation is an ongoing process and community effort involving scientists worldwide.

12. The PGP provides individual sequences of diploid genomes, and results of such projects indicate that the HGP may underestimate genome variation by as much as fivefold. Genome variation between individuals may be 0.5 percent rather than the 0.1 percent estimated from the HGP. Since the PGP provides sequence information on individuals, fundamental questions about human diversity and evolution may be more answerable.

13. Given the speed, efficiency, and recent cost reductions associated with modern sequencing technologies, some scientists believe it is reasonable to expect that 10,000 (10K) vertebrate genomes can be sequenced in 5 years. They believe that such a massive pool of sequences would provide insight into genome evolution and speciation, in addition to providing valuable insight to the human genome through comparative genomics.

14. A number of new subdisciplines of molecular biology will provide the infrastructure for major advances in our understanding of living systems.

The following terms identify specific areas within that infrastructure:

proteomics – proteins in a cell or tissue
metabolomics – enzymatic pathways
glycomics – carbohydrates of a cell or tissue
toxicogenomics – toxic chemicals
metagenomics – environmental issues
pharmacogenomics – customized medicine
transcriptomics – expressed genes

Many other "-omics" are likely in the future.

15. Metagenomics is a relatively new discipline that examines the genomes from entire communities of microbes in environmental samples of water, air, and soil. Virtually every environment on Earth is being sampled in metagenomics projects. A major initiative is a global expedition called the *Sorcerer II* Global Ocean Sampling (GOS) in which researchers travel the globe by yacht and sample as many microbes as possible. Metagenomics is teaching us more about millions of species of microbes, of which only a few thousand have been well characterized. Metagenomics provides new information about genetic diversity in microbes that is important to understanding microbial ecosystems. Metagenomics may also identify genes with novel functions, some of which have potentially valuable applications in medicine and biotechnology.

16. Most microarrays, known also as gene chips, consist of a glass slide that is coated, using a robotic system, with single-stranded DNA molecules. Some microarrays are coated with single-stranded sequences of expressed sequenced tags or DNA sequences that are complementary to gene transcripts. A single microarray can have as many as 20,000 different spots of DNA, each containing a unique sequence. Researchers use microarrays to compare patterns of gene expression in tissues under different conditions or to compare gene expression patterns in normal and diseased tissues. In addition, microarrays can be used to identify pathogens. Microarray databases allow investigators to compare any given pattern to others worldwide.

17. Increased protein production from approximately 20,000 genes is probably related to alternative splicing and various posttranslational processing schemes. In addition, a particular DNA segment may be read in a variety of ways and in two directions.

18. In general, one would expect certain factors (such as heat or salt) to favor evolution to increase

protein stability: distribution of ionic interactions on the surface, density of hydrophobic residues and interactions, and number of hydrogen and disulfide bonds. By examining the codon table, a high GC ratio would favor amino acids Ala, Gly, Pro, Arg, and Trp and minimize the use of Ile, Phe, Lys, Asn, and Tyr. How codon bias influences actual protein stability is not yet understood. Most genomic sequences change by relatively gradual responses to mild selection over long periods of time. They strongly resemble patterns of common descent; that is, they are conserved. Although the same can be said for organisms adapted to extreme environments, extraordinary physiological demands may dictate unexpected sequence bias.

19. Although the β-globin gene family is a relatively large (60kb) sequence and restriction analyses show that it is composed of six genes, one is a pseudogene and therefore does not produce a product. The five functional genes each contain two similarly sized introns, which, when included with noncoding flanking regions (5' and 3') and spacer DNA between genes, account for the 95 percent mentioned in the question.

20. Any time a DNA sequence is conserved in other species, it is likely that sequence has an influence on similar phenotypes. The higher the number of species that conserve the sequence, the higher the likelihood of determining its function. Coupled with mutation analysis and physical mapping, comparative genomics provides a powerful method for linking DNA sequences with complex human diseases.

21. Two factors may be significant in causing a similar gene to function one way in one species and another way in a closely related species. Despite the fact that humans and chimps share significant sequence overlap, there are still approximately 35 million single base differences and about 5 million deletion/addition differences. Such changes influence the molecular environment in which a gene is expressed. Second, the external environment, especially in terms of carbohydrate availability and metabolism, has been different during the evolution of these two species. Such environmental differences may engage a different genetic background (therefore proteome) in which a particular gene is expressed. A protein functioning in one molecular environment may function quite differently in a slightly different environment. Such complexities in gene expression must be addressed when therapies are developed using model organisms.

22. The issue here is whether the organism under consideration is independent and self-reproducing. It appears that the minimum number of genes for a free-living organism is in the range of 250–350. Symbionts can have much smaller genomes and exist with fewer genes because of materials supplied by the host cell. As long as one defines the lifestyle (free-living or symbiont) of the organism in question, it is informative to consider how many genes are needed to accomplish the task of "living."

Chapter 19: Applications and Ethics of Genetic Engineering and Biotechnology

Concept Areas	Corresponding Problems
Genetically Modified Organisms	3
Use of Genetically Engineered Products	2, 4, 5, 6
Genetic Engineering	1, 7, 22
Diagnosing and Screening Genetic Disorders	8, 10, 11, 13
Gene Therapy	1, 14, 15, 16, 17, 18, 21
Genome Analysis	1, 9, 12
DNA Profiling	23
Ethical Issues	2, 3, 5, 19, 20, 21, 22, 23

Structures and Processes Checklist – Significant concepts that deserve special attention are identified with a "*"

(check topic when mastered – provide examples where appropriate – understand the context of each entry)

- ○ **Applications and Ethics**
  - ○ genetic engineering*
  - ○ genetically modified organisms*
  - ○ GMOs
  - ○ biotechnology
- ○ **Genetically Engineered Organisms***
  - ○ biopharmaceutical
  - ○ biopharming
  - ○ insulin production
  - ○ FDA*
  - ○ fusion protein
  - ○ growth hormone
  - ○ transgenic animal hosts*
  - ○ bioreactors
  - ○ biofactories
  - ○ baculovirus
- ○ α-antitrypsin
- ○ antithrombin
- ○ vaccine production*
- ○ edible vaccines
- ○ inactivated vaccines*
- ○ attenuated vaccines*
- ○ subunit vaccine*
- ○ hepatitis B virus
- ○ human papilloma virus
- ○ HPV
- ○ **Genetic Engineering of Plants***
  - ○ selective breeding
  - ○ agricultural biotechnology
  - ○ transgenic crops*
  - ○ herbicide resistance
  - ○ pest resistance

- glyphosate*
- EPSP synthase*
- Bt crops*
- nutritional enhancement*
- golden rice
- **Transgenic Animals***
  - Chinook salmon
  - growth hormone
  - mastitis
  - GloFish
- **Synthetic Genomes***
  - genome transplantation*
  - JCVI*
  - synthetic biology
- **Medical Diagnosis***
  - amniocentesis*
  - chorionic villus sampling*
  - fetal cell sorting
  - restriction enzyme analysis*
  - RFLP
  - sickle-cell anemia
  - allele-specific oligonucleotides*
  - ASOs
  - single-nucleotide polymorphism*
  - SNPs
  - preimplantation genetic diagnosis*
  - PGD
  - DNA microarrays*
  - genome scans*

- CFTR
- field
- **Gene-Expression Microarrays***
  - cDNA*
  - DLBCL
  - genotype analysis of pathogens*
  - SARS*
  - H5N1*
- **Genome-Wide Association***
  - GWAS*
- **Gene Therapy***
  - MLV
  - SCID
  - ADA
  - OTC
  - barriers to gene therapy*
  - adenovirus*
  - viral integrase*
  - target insertion*
- **Gene Editing and Silencing***
  - antisense oligonucleotide*
  - RNA interference*
  - RNAi
- **Ethical, Social, and Legal Issues***
  - GMOs
  - GM foods
- **Genetic Testing***
  - ELSI program*

Chapter 19 Applications and Ethics of Genetic Engineering and Biotechnology

- genetic nondiscrimination*
- direct-to-consumer testing*
- DTC
- Genetic Testing Registry*

- GTR
- DNA and gene patents*
- intellectual property*
- patents and synthetic biology

Answers to Now Solve This

19-1. In many cases, the natural immune system of the host mounts a destructive attack against the introduction of foreign macromolecules. Thus, any injected plasmid or virus might just be negated before it can be effective. In addition, regulating the output of the introduced DNA is difficult. In most cases studied to date, the stability of the injected material and its regulation have been shortcomings.

19-2. The child in question is a carrier of the deletion in the β-globin gene, just as the parents are carriers. Its genotype is therefore $\beta^A\beta^o$.

19-3. It will hybridize by base complementation to the normal DNA sequence.

19-4. (a,b) One of the main problems with gene therapy is delivery of the desired virus to the target tissue in an effective manner. Several of the problems involving the use of retroviral vectors are the following: (1) Integration into the host must be cell specific so as not to damage nontarget cells. (2) Retroviral integration into host cell genomes occurs only if the host cell is replicating. (3) Insertion of the viral genome might influence nontarget, but essential, genes. (4) Retroviral genomes have a low cloning capacity and cannot carry large inserted sequences as are many human genes. (5) There is a possibility that recombination with host viruses will produce an infectious virus that may do harm.

(c) The question posed here plays on the practical versus the ethical. It would certainly be more efficient (although perhaps more difficult technically) to engineer germ tissue, for once it is done in a family, the disease would be eliminated in that family. However, there are considerable ethical problems associated with germ-line therapy. It recalls previous attempts of the eugenics movements of past decades, which involved the use of selective breeding to purify the human stock. Some present-day biologists have said publically that germ-line gene therapy will *not* be conducted.

1. (a) In general, if the modified plant is not toxic or allergenic as determined in test organisms, and no other negative physiological properties have been identified, it is considered safe for human consumption. Potentially harmful agents are usually tested at mega-dose levels to detect potential problems. Protein-based allergenicity is often detected by comparing proteins of transgenic plants with amino acid sequences of known allergens.

(b) Scientists at JCVI introduced a series of marker sequences into JCVI-syn1.0 that were then assayed in the recombinant host.

(c) The RFLP pattern differs between the gene for normal hemoglobin and that for sickle-cell hemoglobin.

(d) Microarrays can be used as platforms on which to hybridize DNA or RNA from various tissues. RNA populations from different tissues, pathological or healthy, will give different patterns of hybridization, a so-called transcriptome analysis.

(e) Genome-wide association studies involve scanning the genomes of thousands of unrelated individuals with a particular disease and compare with individuals who do not have the disease. GWAS attempt to identify genes that influence disease risk.

(f) A number of factors impact the utility of gene therapy. A suitable vector must be selected and properly engineered to carry and deliver the desired product on an appropriate schedule. The vector must be stable yet not trigger an immune response. If the vector is to integrate into the host DNA, it must do so without causing harm.

2. There are concerns about proper testing of GM crops and foods for allergenicity, environmental impact, and the possibility of cross-pollination leading to the contamination of native species. If certain crops become the standard and under the control of a few manufacturers, it is likely that the world's supply of genetic variability might be reduced. Concern would increase if such crops routinely contained antibiotic-resistant genetic markers and genes conferring toxicity to pests. A broader concern is that the design and patenting of crops might allow domination of the world food supply by a few companies.

3. Because of the recent rise in food sensitivities (allergies and adverse reactions), the public should

probably have access to the contents of all foods. GMOs have the potential for possessing suites of gene products that might be atypical for a given food and unless consumers know of that possibility, harm could result. Some argue that consumers have a right to know about GMOs as a matter of principle regardless of potential health risks.

4. In general, bacteria do not process eukaryotic proteins in the same manner as eukaryotes. Transgenic eukaryotes are more likely to correctly process eukaryotic proteins, thus increasing the likelihood of their normal biological activity.

5. From a purely scientific viewpoint, there will be no added danger to consuming cow's milk from cloned animals. However, some individuals may have an aversion to organismic cloning, and supporting such activities through consumption of products of cloned organisms may be viewed negatively on moral grounds. It is likely that public sentiment will pressure for labeling of cloned products on the grounds that consumers should be able to make an informed choice as to the origin of such products.

6. (a) Both the saline and column extracts of Lkt50 appear to be capable of inducing at least 50 percent neutralization of toxicity when injected into rabbits.

(b) In order for a successful edible vaccine to be developed, numerous hurdles must be overcome. The immunogen must be stably incorporated into the host plant hereditary material and the host must express only that immunogen. During feeding, the immunogen must be transported across the intestinal wall unaltered, or altered in such a way as to stimulate the desired immune response. There must be guarantees that potentially harmful byproducts of transgenesis have not been produced. In other words, broad ecological and environmental issues must be addressed to prevent a transgenic plant from becoming an unintended vector for harm to the environment or any organisms feeding on the plant (directly or indirectly).

7. The Venter team compared a number of genomes each with a small number of genes and identified 256 genes that may represent the minimum number of genes for life. They also used transposon-based mutations to determine the number of genes essential for life. Finally, they synthesized short DNA segments and assembled them into a synthetic genome that possessed characteristics of living systems.

8. Even though you have developed a method for screening seven of the mutations described, it is possible that negative results can occur when the person carries the gene for CF. In other words, the specific probes (or allele-specific oligonucleotides) that have been developed will not necessarily be useful for screening all mutant alleles. In addition, the cost-effectiveness of such a screening proposal would need to be considered.

9. A microarray is a solid support containing an orderly arrangement of DNA samples. A typical array contains thousands of DNA spots that may be small oligonucleotides, cDNAs, or short genomic sequences. Labeled sequences hybridize to the immobilized DNAs by standard base pairing. Such technology allows a method for monitoring RNA expression levels of thousands of genes in virtually any cell population. Using microarray technology, researchers can observe the overall behavior of the genome in cancer and normal cells and, by comparison, determine which genes are active or inactive under various circumstances. It is possible to identify the set of genes whose expression or lack thereof defines the properties of each tumor type. This application can, therefore, lead to precise diagnosis and refine possible therapies. In addition, microarray profiling can be used to determine the efficacy of particular therapies. For instance, one can monitor responses to radiation and/or chemotherapy to determine the degree to which cells are responding to a particular cancer treatment.

10. Because both mutations occur in the CF gene, children who possess both alleles will suffer from CF. With both parents heterozygous, each child born will have a 25 percent chance of developing CF.

11. At this point, there is considerable reluctance to allow the open sharing of genetic information among institutions. In general, the establishment of governmental databases containing our most intimate information is viewed with skepticism. It is likely that considerable time and discussion will elapse before such databases are established.

12. Using restriction enzyme analysis to detect point mutations in humans is a tedious trial-and-error process. Given the size of the human genome in terms of base sequences and the relatively low number of

unique restriction enzymes, the likelihood of matching a specific point mutation, separate from other normal sequence variations, to a desired gene is low.

13. Genome-wide association studies involve scanning the genomes of thousands of unrelated individuals with a particular disease and compare the results with those from individuals who do not have the disease. GWAS attempt to identify genes that influence disease risk.

14. As with all therapies, the cure must be less hazardous than the disease. In the case of viral-mediated gene therapy, the antigenicity of the virus must not interfere with the delivery system; such antigenicity can cause inflammation or more severe immunologic responses. Combating the host immune response may involve the use of immunosuppressive drugs or modification of the vector. The duration of desired gene expression at the diseased site is an issue. Short-period expression may require repeated exposure to the vehicle, which may present undesired responses. For some diseases, local gene therapy through inhalation or injection may produce fewer side effects than systemic exposure. Adenoviruses appear to be particularly useful for gene therapy because they can infect nondividing cells and they can accept relatively large amounts of additional DNA (30kb or more).

15. Although some success has been achieved using gene therapy, major questions remain. First, the vectors that deliver the desired gene must not trigger adverse reactions. Second, at present, integration of some vectors is dependent on DNA replication in the host. All cells in the body are therefore not available to integration of some vectors. Third, precise target integration must be achieved to reduce the introduction of new mutations. Fourth, most human genes are large, whereas many vectors in use today can carry only small inserts. Large cargos will be needed to achieve a broad range of therapies. Finally, desired products of the vector should have long-lasting effects, and the vectors themselves must remain incapable of reverting to an infectious virus.

16. p53 and pRB are tumor suppressor proteins and are required by the cell to effectively monitor the cell cycle. Reduction in their activity would diminish normal cell-cycle controls and most likely lead to cancer. It would be especially important if such viral-vectors are intended to treat cancer where cell-cycle control is likely already compromised.

17. In the case of haplo-insufficient mutations, gene therapy holds promise; however, in "gain-of-function" mutations in all probability, the mutant gene's activity or product must be compromised. RNAi strategies may apply more effectively. Addition of a normal gene probably will not help unless it can compete out the mutant gene product.

18. The two major problems described here are common concerns related to genetic engineering. The first is the localization of the introduced DNA into the target tissue and target location in the genome. Inappropriate targeting may have serious consequences. In addition, it is often difficult to control the output of introduced DNA. Genetic regulation is complicated and subject to a number of factors including upstream and downstream signals as well as various posttranscriptional processing schemes. Artificial control of these factors will prove difficult.

19. Certainly, information provided to physicians and patients about genetic testing is a strong point in favor of wide distribution. It would probably be helpful for companies involved in genetic testing to also participate by providing information peculiar to their operations. It would be necessary, however, that any individual results from tests would be held in strict confidence. It would be helpful if pooled statistical data would be available to the public in terms of frequencies of false positives and negatives, as well as population and or geographical distributions.

20. Given the use to which genetic tests are put and their extreme personal nature, it would seem that FDA regulation is one way to decrease the distribution of misinformation that may be vital to individuals and families.

21. The general consensus is that enhancement therapy, much like germ-line therapy, is unacceptable. However, there are circumstances in which enhancement therapy is approved by the U.S. FDA, which permits the use of growth hormone produced by recombinant DNA technology to treat growth-associated disorders. One might argue that enhancement therapy will lead to the transfer of genes (gene therapy) for the same or similar purpose.

22. (a,b) Because a gene is a product of the natural world, it does not conform to section 101 of U.S. patent laws, which govern patentable matter. Because both the direct-to-consumer test for the *BRCA1* and *BRCA2* genes and Venter's "first-ever human made life form" are original in their process or development, they should be patentable.

23. As with any newly introduced technology, the benefits seem straightforward and testimonials from happy customers can be convincing. One might wonder about the specificity of the tests and their accuracy. Is the laboratory doing the tests regulated in any way? How can one challenge a false positive outcome? Will the DNA profiles of the animals be available to law enforcement in the event a pet is involved in some other activity, such as biting or attacking? Some people purchase insurance for their pets. Will DNA profiles be available to insurance companies?

Chapter 20: Developmental Genetics

Concept Areas	Corresponding Problems
Developmental Concepts	1, 2, 3, 23
Differential Transcription in Development	9, 10
Genetics of Embryonic Development	1, 4
Maternal-effect Genes and Body Plans	1, 5, 8, 14, 15, 16
Zygotic Genes and Segment Formation	6, 7, 17, 19
Homeotic and Hox Genes	1, 11, 12, 13, 18, 21
Arabidopsis Development	20, 21
Cell-cell Interactions in C. elegans	1, 22

Structures and Processes Checklist – Significant concepts that deserve special attention are identified with a "*".

(check topic when mastered – provide examples where appropriate – understand the context of each entry)

- **Developmental Concepts**
  - specification
  - determination*
  - differentiation*
- **Evolutionary Conservation***
  - body plan specification*
  - changes in gene expression*
  - cell-cell communication*
- **Genetic Analysis/*Drosophila***
  - *Drosophila* development*
  - syncytium
  - somatic nuclei
  - anterior-posterior orientation*
  - dorsal-ventral orientation*
  - maternal effect genes*
  - zygotic genes*

- segmentation genes*
- gap genes*
- pair-rule genes*
- polarity genes*
- homeotic selector genes*
- *Hox* genes*
- *runt*
- *RUNX2*
- homeotic mutants*
- homeobox*
- 180-bp
- homeodomain*
- spatially ordered cascade*
- human *Hox* genes*
- *Arabidopsis**
- genetic divergence

181

- MADS-box proteins*
- **Cell-cell Interactions***
  - signaling pathways*
  - Notch signaling pathway
- *C. elegans**
- XX hermaphrodites
- XO males
- vulva formation*

F20-1 Illustration of the relationship between determination and differentiation. Determination sets the program that will later be revealed by differentiation. The variable gene activity hypothesis suggests that different sets of genes are transcriptionally active in differentiated cells.

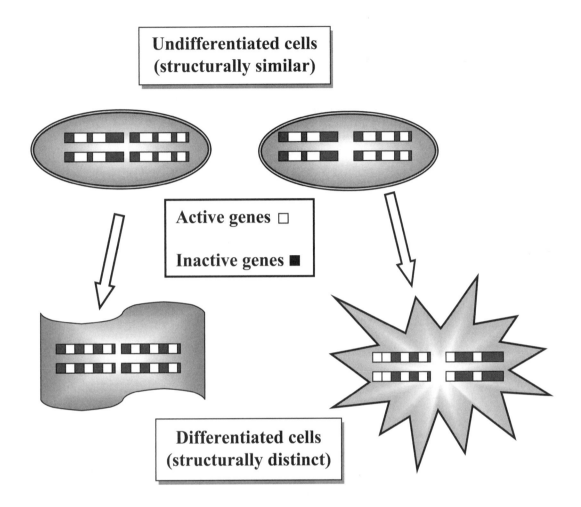

Chapter 20 Developmental Genetics

Answers to Now Solve This

20-1. It is possible that your screen was more inclusive; that is, it identified more subtle alterations than the screen of others. You may have identified several different mutations (multiple alleles) in some of the same genes.

20-2. Because in *ftz/ftz* embryos, the engrailed product is absent and in *en/en* embryos, *ftz* expression is normal, one can conclude that the *ftz* gene product regulates, either directly or indirectly, *en*. Because the *ftz* gene is expressed normally in *en/en* embryos, the product of the *engrailed* gene does not regulate expression of *ftz*.

20-3. Because *her-1⁻* mutations cause males to develop into hermaphrodites, and *tra-1⁻* mutations cause hermaphrodites to develop into males, one may hypothesize that the *her-1⁺* gene produces a product that suppresses hermaphrodite development, whereas the *tra-1⁺* gene product is needed for hermaphrodite development.

Chapter 20 Developmental Genetics

Solutions to Problems and Discussion Questions

1. (a) In general, mutations provide the window for looking at the structure and function of genes. A number of mutant screens have identified hundreds of genes that influence development. Saturational mutagenesis provides an estimate of the lower limit of genes regulating a particular aspect of development.

(b) Our initial understanding of molecular gradients was based on the discovery of mutations that upset those gradients and alter development. Using a variety of labeling techniques, scientists have described egg gradients at the molecular level.

(c) Homeotic selector genes influence clusters of other genes involved in the specification of body parts. Mutations in these genes alter the developmental program in very specific, dramatic ways and have been strikingly apparent to investigators.

(d) In *C. elegans,* specific genes are known to function precisely in vulval development. Mutations in these genes cause abnormal vulval development with eventual cellular development dependent on a cascade of genetic events. Mutational analysis revealed such interactions.

2. *Determination* refers to early developmental and regulatory events that set eventual patterns of gene activity. Determination is not the end result of the regulatory activity; rather, it is the process by which the developmental fate of a particular cell type is fixed. *Differentiation*, on the other hand, follows determination and is the manifestation, in terms of genetic, physiological, and morphological changes, of the determined state.

3. The fact that nuclei from almost any source remain transcriptionally and translationally active substantiates the fact that the genetic code and the ancillary processes of transcription and translation are compatible throughout the animal and plant kingdoms. Because the egg represents an isolated, "closed" system that can be mechanically, environmentally, and to some extent biochemically manipulated, various conditions may be developed that allow one to study facets of gene regulation. For instance, the influence of transcriptional enhancers and suppressors may be studied along with factors that impact translational and post-translational processes. Combinations of injected nuclei may reveal nuclear-nuclear interactions, which could not normally be studied by other methods.

4. The syncytial blastoderm is formed as nuclei migrate to the egg's outer margin or cortex, where additional divisions take place. Plasma membranes organize around each of the nuclei at the cortex, thus creating the cellular blastoderm.

5. (a) Genes that control early development are often dependent on the deposition of their products (mRNA, transcription factors, various structural proteins, etc.) in the egg by the mother. When observable, these are maternal-effect genes.

(b) They are made in the early oocyte or nurse cells during oogenesis.

(c) Such maternal effect genes control early developmental events such as defining anterior-posterior polarity. Such products are placed in eggs during oogenesis and are activated immediately after fertilization.

(d) A variety of phenotypes are possible, and they are often revealed in the offspring of females. Maternal effects reveal the genotype of the mother.

6. (a,b) Zygotic genes are activated or repressed depending on their response to maternal-effect gene products. Three subsets of zygotic genes divide the embryo into segments. These segmentation genes are normally transcribed in the developing embryo, and their mutations have embryonic lethal phenotypes.

(c) The maternal genotype contains zygotic genes, and these are passed to the embryo as with any other gene.

7. The three main classes of zygotic genes are (1) *gap* genes, which specify adjacent segments; (2) *pair-rule* genes, which specify every other segment and a part of each segment; and (3) *segment polarity* genes, which specify homologous parts of each segment.

8. Because the polar cytoplasm contains information to form germ cells, one would expect such a transplantation procedure to generate germ cells in the anterior region. Work done by Illmensee and Mahowald in 1974 verified this expectation.

9. There are several somewhat indirect methods for determining transcriptional activity of a given gene in different cell types. First, if protein products of a given gene are present in different cell types, it can be assumed that the responsible gene is being transcribed. Second, if one is able to actually observe, microscopically, gene activity, as is the case in some specialized chromosomes (polytene chromosomes), gene activity can be inferred by the presence of localized chromosomal puffs. A more direct and common practice to assess transcription of particular genes is to use labeled probes. If a labeled probe can be obtained that contains base sequences that are complementary to the transcribed RNA, then such probes will hybridize to that RNA if present in different tissues. This technique is called *in situ* hybridization and is a powerful tool in the study of gene activity during development.

10. There are a variety of approaches to determine the level of control of a particular gene. First, one may determine whether levels of hnRNA are consistent among various cell types of interest. This is often accomplished by either direct isolation of the RNA and assessment by northern blotting or by use of *in situ* hybridization. If the hnRNA pools for a given gene are consistent in various cell types, then transcriptional control can be eliminated as a possibility. Support for translational control can be achieved directly by determining, in different cell types, the presence of a variety of mRNA species with common sequences. This can be accomplished only when sufficient knowledge exists for specific mRNA trapping or labeling. Clues as to translational control *via* alternative splicing can sometimes be achieved by examining the amino acid sequence of proteins. Similarities in certain structural/functional motifs may indicate alternative RNA processing.

11. *Hox* genes in the *Drosophila* genome can be found in two clusters on chromosome 3: Antp-C and BX-C. They have two properties in common: encoding of transcription factors and colinear gene expression. A *homeotic gene* alters the identity of a segment or field within a segment. All homeotic genes are not *Hox* genes.

12. A dominant gain-of-function mutation is one that changes the specificity or expression pattern of a gene or gene product. The gain-of-function *Antp* mutation causes the wild-type *Antennapedia* gene to be expressed in the eye-antenna disc, and mutant flies have legs on the head in place of antenna.

13. Many of the appendages of the head, including the mouth parts and the antennae, are evolutionary derivatives of ancestral leg structures. In *spineless aristapedia,* the distal portion of the antenna is replaced by its ancestral counterpart, the distal portion of the leg (tarsal segments). Because the replacement of the arista (end of the antenna) can occur by a mutation in a single gene, one would consider that one "selector" gene distinguishes aristal from tarsal structures. Notice that a "one-step" change is involved in the interchange of leg and antennal structures.

14. Because of the regulatory nature of *homeotic* genes in fundamental cellular activities of determination and differentiation, it would be difficult to ignore their possible impact on oncogenesis. Homeotic genes encode DNA binding domains, which influence gene expression and any factor that influences gene expression may, under some circumstances, influence cell cycle control. However attractive this model, there have been no homeotic transformations noted in mammary glands, so the typical expression of mutant homeotic genes in insects is not revealed in mammary tissue according to Lewis (2000). A substantial number of experiments will be needed to establish a functional link between homeotic gene mutation and cancer induction. Mutagenesis and transgenesis experiments are likely to be most productive in establishing a cause-effect relationship.

15. Two coupled approaches might be used. First, one could make transgenic flies that contain a series of deletions spanning all segments of the *bicoid* mRNA: the coding region and 5' and 3' untranslated regions. Comparison of stabilities of individual, deleted mRNAs with controls would indicate whether a particular segment of the mRNA contains a degradation signal sequence. If a degradation-sensitive region or signal sequence is located by deletion, that same intact region, when ligated to a non-involved, nondegraded mRNA (like a ribosomal protein or tubulin mRNA) should foster degradation in a manner similar to the *bicoid* mRNA. If the mRNA from the anterior end of the egg is placed in the posterior of another egg, one could ask if the degradation process is comparable.

16. First, it would be interesting to know whether inhibitors of mitochondrial-ribosomal translation would interfere with germ cell formation. Second, one should know what types of mRNAs are being translated with these ribosomes.

17.

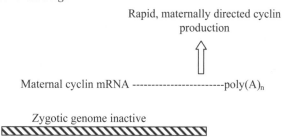

Pre-cell-cycle remodeling:

Rapid, maternally directed cyclin production

Maternal cyclin mRNA ---------------------poly(A)$_n$

Zygotic genome inactive

Post-cell-cycle remodeling:

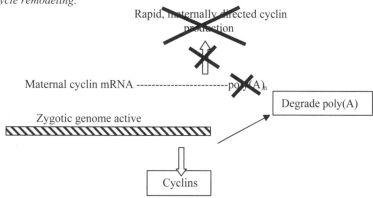

Rapid, maternally directed cyclin production

Maternal cyclin mRNA ---------------------poly(A)$_n$

Zygotic genome active

Degrade poly(A)

Cyclins

18. Given the information in the problem, it is likely that this gene normally controls the expression of *BX-C* genes in all body segments. The wild-type product of *esc* stored in the egg may be required to interpret the information correctly stored in the egg cortex.

19. (a) The term "rescued" is often used when the introduction of genes from an outside source (within or among species) restores the wild-type phenotype from a mutant organism.

(b) Results such as these, and there are many like them, indicate the extreme conservation of protein structure and function across phylogenetically distant organisms. Such results attest to the conservation from a distant common ancestor of fundamental molecular species during development. Failure to adhere to a common developmental theme is rewarded by death.

20. Three classes of flower *homeotic* genes are known that are activated in an overlapping pattern to specify various floral organs. Class *A* genes give rise to sepals. Expression of *A* and *B* class genes specify petals, *B* and *C* genes control stamen formation, and expression of *C* genes gives rise to carpels.

21. The *Polycomb* gene family induces changes in chromatin that influence *Hox* gene expression. A gene in *Arabidopsis* has significant homology to the *Polycomb* gene family and also works by altering chromatin structure. The cross reactivity is thus related to the Polycomb product's effect on chromatin. Such parallel functions indicate that mechanisms of regulation are conserved over vast evolutionary distances.

22. If the *her-1*$^+$ product acts as a negative regulator, then when the gene is mutant, suppression over *tra-1*$^+$ is lost, and hermaphroditism would be the result. This hypothesis fits the information provided. The double mutant should be male because even though there is no suppression from *her-1*$^-$, there is no *tra-1*$^+$ product to support hermaphrodite development.

23. (a,b) A number of studies indicate that genes in *Drosophila* have evolutionary counterparts (orthologs) in other organisms, including humans. A number of similar genes influence eye development in both insects and vertebrates. Genes that produce eyes are part of a complex network of at least seven genes that constitute the master regulators of eye development. Each gene functions in coordination with others in a conserved network that is used by broad evolutionary groups. Such genes, descended from common ancestral genes that have the same function in different species, are called orthologs.

(c) Because development is dependent on the coordinated output of numerous genes, genetic networks are probably the rule rather than the exception. The fact that a single genetic change (in the case of the mouse homolog of the fly *eyeless* gene) can trigger the formation of ectopic eyes in *Drosophila* shows that major components of developmental networks may be evolutionarily conserved. Another example of a regulatory network involves vulval development in *C. elegans*.

Chapter 21: Quantitative Genetics and Multifactorial Traits

Concept Areas	Corresponding Problems
Phenotypic Expression	10, 15, 22
Continuous Variation and Polygenes	1, 2, 3
Genetic Basis	4, 5, 6, 7, 20, 21
Heritability	1, 3, 9, 12, 13, 15, 16, 17, 18, 19
Mapping	23
Statistics	11, 14
Twin Studies	1, 3, 8

Structures and Processes Checklist – Significant concepts that deserve special attention are identified with a "∗".

(check topic when mastered – provide examples where appropriate – understand the context of each entry)

- **Quantitative Genetics**
  - quantitative inheritance*
  - polygenes*
  - multifactorial
  - complex traits
- **Quantitative Traits**
  - multiple-factor*
  - multiple-gene
  - additive allele*
  - nonadditive allele*
  - continuous variation*
  - number of polygenes*
- **Statistical Analysis**
  - normal distribution*
  - mean*
  - central tendency*

- variance*
- standard deviation*
- standard error*
- covariance
- heritability values*
- heritability
- phenotypic variance*
- genotypic variance*
- environmental variance*
- genotype-environment interaction*
- broad-sense heritability*
- narrow-sense heritability*
- additive variance
- dominance variance
- interactive variance
- artificial selection

- selection response
- selection differential
- **Twin Studies***
  - monozygotic twins*
  - identical twins
  - dizygotic twins*
  - fraternal twins
  - concordant*
  - discordant*
- limitations of twin studies
- copy number variation
- somatic mosaicism
- epigenetics*
- QTL mapping*
- quantitative trait locus
- DNA markers*
- expression QTLs
- protein QTLs

Chapter 21 Quantitative Genetics and Multifactorial Traits

Answers to Now Solve This

21-1. (a) Because 1/256 of the F_2 plants are 20 cm and 1/256 are 40 cm, there must be 4 gene pairs involved in determining flower size.

(b) Because there are nine size classes, one can conduct the following backcross:

AaBbCcDd × *AABBCCDD*

The frequency distribution in the backcross would be:

1/16	=	40 cm
4/16	=	37.5 cm
6/16	=	35 cm
4/16	=	32.5 cm
1/16	=	30 cm

21-2. (a) Taking the sum of the values and dividing by the number in the sample gives the following means

mean sheep fiber length = 7.7 cm   *mean fleece weight* = 6.4 kg

The variance for each is

variance sheep fiber length = 6.097   *variance fleece weight* = 3.12

The standard deviation is the square root of the variance:

sheep fiber length = 2.469   *fleece weight* = 1.766

(b,c) The covariance for the two traits is 30.36/7, or 4.34, whereas the correlation coefficient is +0.998.

(d) There is a very high correlation between fleece weight and fiber length, and it is likely that this correlation is not by chance. Even though correlation does not mean cause and effect, it would seem logical that as you increased fiber length, you would also increase fleece weight. It is probably safe to say that the increase in fleece weight is directly related to an increase in fiber length.

21-3. The role of genetics and the role of the environment can be studied by comparing the expression of traits in monozygotic and dizygotic twins. The higher concordance value for monozygotic twins as compared with the value for dizygotic twins indicates a significant genetic component for a given trait. Notice that for traits including blood type, eye color, and mental retardation, there is a fairly significant difference between MZ and DZ groups. However, for measles, the difference is not as significant, indicating a greater role of the environment. Hair color has a significant genetic component, as do idiopathic epilepsy, schizophrenia, diabetes, allergies, cleft lip, and club foot. The genetic component to mammary cancer is present but minimal according to these data.

191

Solutions to Problems and Discussion Questions

1. (a) The number of polygenes involved in a polygenic trait can often be estimated by solving for *n* in the formula if the ratio of F_2 individuals resembling either of the two extreme P_1 phenotypes can be determined.

$$1/4^n$$

It is also possible to estimate the number of polygenes using the $(2n + 1)$ rule, where $(2n + 1)$ is the number of possible phenotypes, and *n* equals the number of additive loci.

(b) The multiple factor hypothesis was originally based on experiment results involving pigmentation in wheat. Such results showed that a number of additive alleles acting in Mendelian fashion could explain continuous variation.

(c) When a number of parameters are known, environmental impact on a quantitatively inherited trait is often assessed by heritability estimates (broad and narrow sense). Using highly inbred strains of plants and animals reared under varying conditions and twin studies in humans are helpful in determining the environmental impact on traits.

(d) Differences in inherited disease states indicate that copy number variation and epigenetics alter the genotypes of all individuals including monozygotic twins.

2. In *discontinuous* variation, the influences of each gene pair are not additive, and more typical Mendelian ratios such as 9:3:3:1 and 3:1 result. In *continuous* variation, different gene pairs interact (usually additively) to produce a phenotype that is less "stepwise" in distribution. Inheritance involving polygenic systems follows a more continuous distribution.

3. (a) *Polygenes* are those genes that are involved in determining continuously varying or multiple factor traits.

(b) *Additive alleles* are those alleles that account for the hereditary influence on the phenotype in an additive way.

(c) *Monozygotic twins* are derived from a single fertilized egg and are thus genetically identical to each other. They provide a method for determining the influence of genetics and environment on certain traits. *Dizygotic twins* arise from two eggs fertilized

by two sperm cells. They have the same genetic relationship as siblings.

The role of genetics and the role of the environment can be studied by comparing the expression of traits in monozygotic and dizygotic twins. The higher concordance value for monozygotic twins as compared with the value for dizygotic twins indicates a significant genetic component for a given trait.

(d) *Heritability* is a measure of the degree to which the phenotypic variation of a given trait is due to genetic factors. A high heritability indicates that genetic factors are major contributors to phenotypic variation, whereas environmental factors have little impact.

(e) QTL stands for Quantitative Trait Loci, which are situations in which multiple genes contribute to a quantitative trait.

4. If you add the numbers given for the ratio, you obtain the value of 16, which is indicative of a dihybrid cross. The distribution is that of a dihybrid cross with additive effects.

(a) Because a dihybrid result has been identified, there are two loci involved in the production of color. There are two alleles at each locus for a total of four alleles.

(b,c) Because the description of red, medium red, and so on, gives us no indication of a *quantity* of color in any form of units, we would not be able to actually quantify a unit amount for each change in color. We can say that each gene (additive allele) provides an equal unit amount to the phenotype, and the colors differ from each other in multiples of that unit amount. The number of additive alleles needed to produce each phenotype is given next:

1/16	=	dark red	=	*AABB*
4/16	=	medium-dark red	=	2*AABb*
				2*AaBB*
6/16	=	medium red	=	*AAbb*
				4*AaBb*
				aaBB
4/16	=	light red	=	2*aaBb*
				2*Aabb*
1/16	=	white	=	*aabb*

(d)

F_1 = all light red
F_2 = 1/4 medium red
    2/4 light red
    1/4 white

5. (a) It is *possible* that two parents of moderate height can produce offspring that are much taller or shorter than either parent because segregation can produce a variety of gametes as follows:

rrSsTtuu × *RrSsTtUu*
(moderate)   (moderate)

Offspring from this cross can range from very tall *RrSSTTUu* (14 "tall" units) to very short *rrssttuu* (8 "small" units).

(b) If the individual with a minimum height, *rrssttuu*, is married to an individual of intermediate height, *RrSsTtUu*, the offspring can be no taller than the height of the tallest parent. Notice that there is no way of having more than four uppercase alleles in the offspring.

6. As you read this question, notice that the strains are inbred, therefore homozygous, and that approximately 1/250 represents the shortest and tallest groups in the F_2 generation. See $1/4^n$ formula in the text.

(a,b) Referring to the text, see that where four gene pairs act additively, the proportion of one of the extreme phenotypes to the total number of offspring is 1/256. The same may be said for the other extreme type. The extreme types in this problem are the 12cm and 36cm plants. From this observation, one would suggest that there are four gene pairs involved.

(c) If there are four gene pairs, there are nine ($2n + 1$) phenotypic categories and eight increments between these categories. Because there is a difference of 24cm between the extremes, 24cm/8 = 3cm for each increment (each of the additive alleles).

(d) A typical F_1 cross that produces a "typical" F_2 distribution would be one in which all gene pairs are heterozygous (*AaBbCcDd*), independently assorting, and additive. There are many possible sets of parents that would give an F_1 of this type. The limitation is that each parent has genotypes that give a height of 24cm as stated in the problem. Because the parents are inbred, it is expected that they are fully homozygous. An example:

AABBccdd × *aabbCCDD*

(e) Because the *aabbccdd* genotype gives a height of 12cm and each uppercase allele adds 3cm to the height, there are many possibilities for an 18cm plant:

AAbbccdd,

AaBbccdd,

aaBbCcdd, and so on.

Any plant with seven uppercase letters will be 33cm tall:

AABBCCDd,

AABBCcDD,

AABbCCDD, for example.

7. (a) There is a fairly continuous range of "quantitative" phenotypes in the F_2 and an F_1 that is between the phenotypes of the two parents; therefore, one can conclude that some phenotypic blending is occurring that is probably the result of several gene pairs acting in an additive fashion. Because the extreme phenotypes (6cm and 30cm) each represent 1/64 of the total, it is likely that there are three gene pairs in this cross. Remember, trihybrid crosses that show independent assortment of genes have a denominator (4^3) of 64 in ratios. Also, the fact that there are seven categories of phenotypes, which, because of the relationship $2n + 1 = 7$, would give the number of gene pairs (n) of 3. The genotypes of the parents would be combinations of alleles that would produce a 6cm (*aabbcc*) tail and a 30cm (*AABBCC*) tail, WHEREAS the 18cm offspring would have a genotype of *AaBbCc*.

(b) A mating of an *AaBbCc* (for example) pig with the 6cm *aabbcc* pig would result in the following offspring:

Gametes (18 cm tail)	Gamete (6 cm tail)	Offspring
ABC		AaBbCc (18 cm)
ABc		AaBbcc (14 cm)
AbC		AabbCc (14 cm)
Abc	abc	Aabbcc (10 cm)
aBC		aaBbCc (14 cm)
aBc		aaBbcc (10 cm)
abC		aabbCc (10 cm)
abc		aabbcc (6 cm)

In this example, a 1:3:3:1 ratio is the result. However, had a different 18cm TAILED PIG been selected, a different ratio would occur:

AABbcc × *aabbcc*

Gametes (18 cm tail)	Gamete (6 cm tail)	Offspring
ABc	*abc*	*AaBbcc* (14 cm)
Abc		*Aabbcc* (10 cm)

8. For height, notice that average differences between MZ twins reared together (1.7 cm) and those MZ twins reared apart (1.8 cm) are similar (meaning little environmental influence) and considerably less than differences of DZ twins (4.4cm) or sibs (4.5) reared together. These data indicate that genetics plays a major role in determining height.

However, for weight, notice that MZ twins reared together have a much smaller (1.9 kg) difference than MZ twins reared apart, indicating that the environment has a considerable impact on weight. By comparing the weight differences of MZ twins reared apart with DZ twins and sibs reared together, one can conclude that the environment has almost as much an influence on weight as genetics.

For ridge count, the differences between MZ twins reared together and those reared apart are small. For the data in the table, it would appear that ridge count and height have the highest heritability values.

9. Comparison of phenotypic variances between monozygotic and dizygotic traits provides an estimate of broad-sense heritability (H^2).

10. Many traits, especially those we view as quantitative, are likely to be determined by a polygenic mode with possible environmental influences. The following are some common examples: height, general body structure, skin color, and perhaps most common behavioral traits including intelligence.

11. At first glance, this problem looks as if it will be an arithmetic headache; however, the problem can be simplified.

(a) The mean is computed by adding the measurements of all of the individuals, then dividing by the number of individuals. In this case, there are 760 corn plants. To keep from having to add 760 numbers, merely multiply each height group by the number of individuals in each group. Add all the products, then divide by *n* (760). This gives a value for the mean of 140cm.

(b) For the variance, use the formula given here (as in the text):

$$s^2 = V = n\Sigma f(x^2) - (\Sigma fx)^2 / n(n-1)$$

To simplify the calculations, determine the square of each height group (100cm, for example), then multiply the value by the number in each group.

For the first group (100cm), we would have:

$$100 \times 100 \times 20 = 200000$$

The rest of the groups are as follows:

$110 \times 110 \times 60$	= 726000
$120 \times 120 \times 90$	= 1296000
$130 \times 130 \times 130$	= 2197000
$140 \times 140 \times 180$	= 3528000
$150 \times 150 \times 120$	= 2700000
$160 \times 160 \times 70$	= 1792000
$170 \times 170 \times 50$	= 1445000
$180 \times 180 \times 40$	= 1296000
	= 15180000

Now, the mean squared, multiplied by *n* is as follows:

$$140 \times 140 \times 760 = 14896000$$

Completing the calculations gives the following:

$$(15180000 - 14896000)/759$$
$$= 284000/759$$

$$s^2 = V = 374.18$$

(c) The *standard deviation* is the square root of the variance or 19.34.

(d) The *standard error* of the mean is the standard deviation divided by the square root of *n*, or about 0.70. The plot approximates a normal distribution. Variation is continuous.

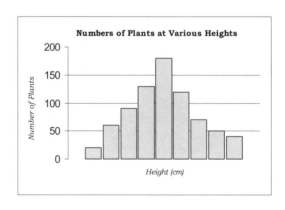

12. (a) Using the following equations, H^2 and h^2 can be calculated as follows.

For back fat:

Broad-sense heritability = H^2 = 12.2/30.6 = 0.398
Narrow-sense heritability = h^2 = 8.44/30.6 = 0.276

For body length:

Broad-sense heritability = H^2 = 26.4/52.4 = 0.504

Narrow-sense heritability = h^2 = 11.7/52.4 = 0.223

(b) For a trait that is quantitatively measured, the relative importance of genetic *versus* environmental factors may be formally assessed by examining the heritability index (H^2 or broad heritability). In animal and plant breeding, a measure of potential response to selection based on additive variance and dominance variance is termed narrow-sense heritability (h^2). A relatively high narrow-sense heritability is a prediction of the impact selection may have in altering an initial randomly breeding population. Therefore, of the two traits, selection for back fat would produce more response.

13. The formula for estimating heritability is

$$H^2 = V_G / V_P$$

where V_G and V_P are the genetic and phenotypic components of variation, respectively. The main issue in this question is obtaining some estimate of two components of phenotypic variation: genetic and environmental. V_P is the combination of genetic and environmental variance. Because the two parental strains are inbred, they are assumed to be homozygous and the variances of 4.2 and 3.8 are considered to be the result of environmental influences. The average of these two values is 4.0. The F_1 is also genetically homogeneous and gives us an additional estimation of the environmental factors.

By averaging with the parents

$$[(4.0 + 5.6)/2 = 4.8]$$

we obtain a relatively good idea of environmental impact on the phenotype. The phenotypic variance in the F_2 is the sum of the genetic (V_G) and environmental (V_E) components. We have estimated the environmental input as 4.8, so 10.3 (V_P) minus 4.8 gives us an estimate of (V_G), which is 5.5. Heritability then becomes 5.5/10.3 or 0.53. This value, when viewed in percentage form indicates that about 53 percent of the variation in plant height is due to genetic influences.

14. (a) For vitamin A:

$$h_A{}^2 = V_A/V_P = V_A/(V_E + V_A + V_D) = 0.097$$

For cholesterol: $h_A{}^2 = 0.223$

(b) Cholesterol content should be influenced to a greater extent by selection.

15. Given that both narrow-sense heritability values are relatively high, it is likely that a farmer would be able to alter both milk protein content and butterfat by selection. The value of 0.91 for the correlation coefficient between protein content and butterfat suggests that if one selects for butterfat, protein content will increase. However, correlation coefficients describe the extent to which variation in one quantitative trait is associated with variation in another and does not reveal the underlying causes of such variation. Assuming that these dairy cows had been selected for high butterfat in the past and increased protein content followed that selection (for butterfat), it is likely that selection for butterfat would continue to correlate with increased protein content. However, there may well be a point where physiological circumstances change and selection for high butterfat may be at the expense of protein content.

16. $h^2 = (7.5 - 8.5/6.0 - 8.5) = 0.4$

(realized heritability)

17. Given the realized heritability value of 0.4, it is unlikely that selection experiments would cause a rapid and/or significant response to selection. A minor response might result from intense selection.

18. $h^2 = 0.3 = (M_2 - 60/80 - 60)$

$$M_2 = 66 \text{ grams}$$

19. Because the rice plants are genetically identical, V_G is zero and $H^2 = V_G/V_P$ = zero. Broad-sense heritability is a measure to which the phenotypic variance is due to genetic factors. In this case, with genetically identical plants, H^2 is zero, and the variance observed in grain yield is due to the environment. Selection would not be effective in this strain of rice.

20. The best way to approach this problem is to first determine the number of gene pairs involved. Notice that all the F_1 plants are uniform and are in the middle of the extremes of 3" and 15"; therefore the parents must each be homozygous and at the extremes. Notice also that there are 13 classes in the F_2, so there must be six gene pairs. See the text for an explanation of the $2n + 1$ formula.

(a) There are two ways to answer this section, a hard way and an easy way. The hard way would to take a big sheet of paper, make the cross (*AaBbCcDdEeFf* × *AaBbCcDdEeFf*), collect the genotypes, and calculate the ratios.

This method would be very laborious and error-prone. The easy way would be to re-read the material on the binomial expansion and note the pattern preceding each expression. Notice that all numbers other than the 1's are equal to the sum of the two numbers directly above them. By enlarging the numbers to include six gene pairs, you can arrive at the 13 classes and their frequencies:

3" = 1	4" = 12	5" = 66
6" = 220	7" = 495	8" = 792
9" = 924	10" = 792	11" = 495
12" = 220	13" = 66	14" = 12
15" = 1		

To check your calculations, be certain that your frequencies total 4096. You will also notice an additional shortcut in that because the distribution is symmetrical, you need only calculate to the center and the remainder will be in the reverse order.

(b) To determine the outcome of a cross of the F_1 plants in the test cross, apply the formula that allows you to calculate any set of components: $n!/(s!t!)$ where n = total number of events (6), s = number of events of outcome a and t = number of events of outcome b. For example, to determine how many 6" plants would be recovered from the cross *AaBbCcDdEeFf* × *aabbccddeeff*, we are really asking how many will have three additive alleles (uppercase) and three non-additive alleles (lowercase).

$$6!/(3!3!) = 20$$

Applying this formula throughout gives the following frequencies:

3" = 1	4" = 6	5" = 15
6" = 20	7" = 15	8" = 6
9" = 1		

The total is 64. You can check your logic by considering that there should be only 1/64 with no additive alleles (3") and 1/64 with all additive alleles (9").

21. The solution to these types of problems rests on determining the ratio of individuals expressing the extreme phenotype to the total number of individuals. In this case, 8:2028 is equal to 1:253, which is close to 1:256. Note that the value of 2028 is used in this calculation because *both* extreme offspring numbers are used. If there are three gene pairs, the ratio is 1:64, four gene pairs 1:256, or five gene pairs 1:1024. Therefore, these data indicate that there are four gene pairs that influence size in these guinea pigs.

22. The level of blood sugar varies considerably from individual to individual, day to day, and hour to hour, and on a population level, it displays continuous variation. However, the diagnosis of Type II diabetes is set by relatively fixed criteria. A fasting blood sugar level of 126 mg/dL or higher, repeated on different days, is diagnostic of diabetes. A casual (non-fasting) blood sugar level of 200 mg/dL or higher is suggestive of diabetes. In either case, although the level of blood sugar is influenced by a variety of factors (polygenic and environmental), the actual diagnosis of the disease leads one to be classified as diabetic or not diabetic. Because there are only two phenotypic classes (or three if one included the prediabetic state), diabetes is referred to as a threshold trait.

23. (a,b) In many instances, a trait may be clustered in families, yet, traditional mapping procedures may not be applicable because the trait might be influenced by a number of genes. In general, researchers look for associations to particular DNA sequences (molecular markers). When the trait cosegregates with a particular maker and it statistically associates with that trait above chance, a likely QTL has been identified. Markers such as RFLPs, SNPs, and microsatellites are often used because they are highly variable, relatively easy to assess, and present in all individuals.

Chapter 22: Population and Evolutionary Genetics

Concept Areas	Corresponding Problems
Variation	1
Sequence Analysis	1, 2, 3, 5, 22
Hardy–Weinberg Computations	6, 7, 9, 11, 12, 13, 14, 15
Hardy–Weinberg Assumptions	1, 8, 10, 19
Speciation	1, 4, 16, 20, 21, 22, 23, 25
Mutation	17, 18
Gene Therapy	24

Structures and Processes Checklist – Significant concepts that deserve special attention are identified with a "*".

(check topic when mastered – provide examples where appropriate – understand the context of each entry)

- **Population Genetics**
    - evolutionary aspects*
    - speciation*
    - microevolution
    - macroevolution
- **Genetic Variation Is Present***
    - population*
    - gene pool*
    - detecting genetic variation*
    - artificial selection*
    - nucleotide sequences*
    - cystic fibrosis
    - CFTR
- **Hardy–Weinberg Law***
    - ideal population
    - infinitely large*
    - random mating*

- no mutation*
- no migration*
- no selection*
- genic frequencies*
- genotypic frequencies*
- H-W equation*
- genetic variability
- **H-W in Human Populations***
    - examples*
    - testing the H-W equilibrium*
    - multiple alleles*
    - ABO blood groups*
- **Natural Selection***
    - genetic variation*
    - variations heritable*
    - exponential reproduction*
    - struggle for survival*

- detecting natural selection*
- fitness and selection*
- types of selection
- directional selection*
- stabilizing selection*
- disruptive selection*
- **Mutation Creates New Alleles***
  - mutation rates*
- **Migration and Gene Flow***
  - calculations*
- **Genetic Drift***
  - founder effect*
  - genetic bottleneck*
  - examples*
- **Nonrandom Mating***
  - positive assertive mating*
  - negative assertive mating*
  - inbreeding*
  - coefficient of inbreeding*
  - *F*

- **Reduced Gene Flow***
  - species*
  - genetic divergence*
  - reproductive isolating mechanisms
  - prezygotic isolating mechanisms*
  - postzygotic isolating mechanisms*
  - speciation*
  - rate of macroevolution*
- **Phylogeny***
  - node
  - phylogenetic trees*
  - amino acid sequences
  - cytochrome c
  - genetic equidistance*
  - minimal mutational distance*
  - molecular clocks*
  - genomics
  - molecular evolution*
  - genetic divergence
  - Neanderthals and humans*

F22-1 Simple illustration of the relationships among populations, individuals, alleles, and allelic frequencies (*p* and *q*).

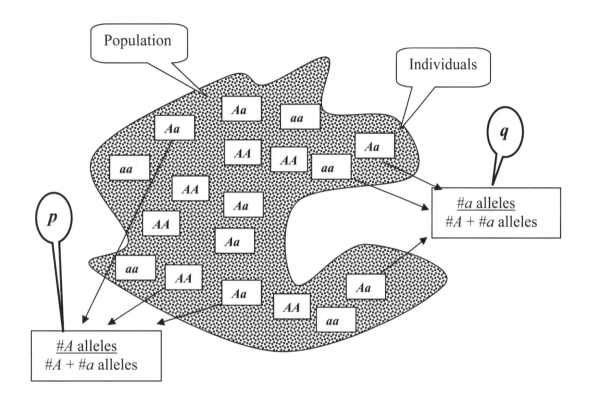

F22-2 Diagram of the relationships among inbreeding, heterosis, and homozygosity. Note that as inbreeding occurs, heterosis decreases and homozygosity increases.

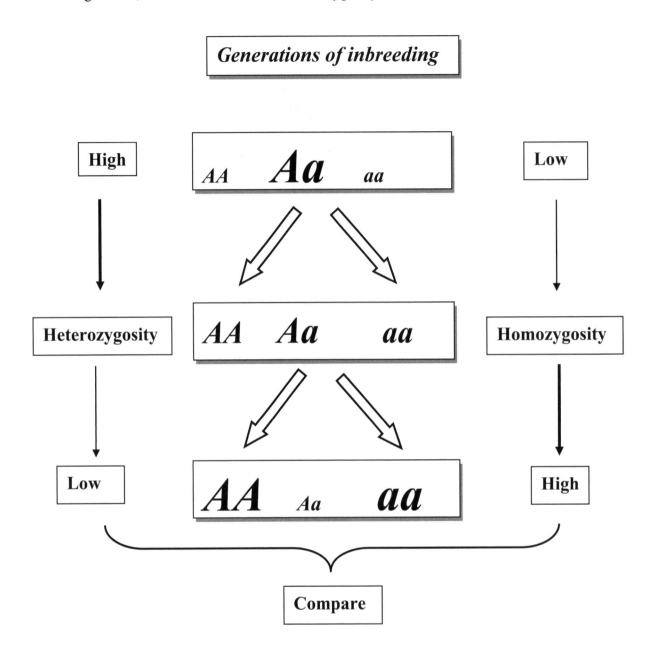

Chapter 22 Population and Evolutionary Genetics

Answers to Now Solve This

22-1. Because the alleles follow a dominant/recessive mode, one can use the equation $\sqrt{q^2}$ to calculate q, from which all other aspects of the answer depend. The frequency of aa types is determined by dividing the number of nontasters (37) by the total number of individuals (125).

$q^2 = 37/125 = 0.296$
$q = 0.544$
$p = 1 - q$
$p = 0.456$

The frequencies of the genotypes are determined by applying the formula $p^2 + 2pq + q^2$ as follows:

Frequency of AA $= p^2$
$= (0.456)^2$
$= 0.208$ or 20.8%

Frequency of Aa $= 2pq$
$= 2(0.456)(0.544)$
$= 0.496$ or 49.6%

Frequency of aa $= q^2$
$= (0.544)^2$
$= 0.296$ or 29.6%

When completing such a set of calculations, it is a good practice to add the final percentages to be certain that they total 100 percent. (Note that calculation requires the assumption that this population is in Hardy–Weinberg equilibrium with respect to the gene for PTC tasting.)

22-2. (a) For the CCR5 analysis, first determine p and q. With the frequencies of all the genotypes, one can add 0.6 and 0.351/2 to provide p ($= 0.7755$); q will be 0.049 and 0.351/2 = 0.2245

The equilibrium values will be as follows:

Frequency of l/l $= p^2$ $= (0.7755)^2 = 0.6014$ or 60.14%

Frequency of $l/\Delta32$ $= 2pq$ $= 2(0.7755)(0.2245) = 0.3482$ or 34.82%

Frequency of $\Delta32/\Delta32$ $= q^2$ $= (0.2245)^2 = 0.0504$ or 5.04%

Comparing these equilibrium values with the observed values strongly suggests that the observed values are drawn from a population in Hardy–Weinberg equilibrium.

(b) For the AS (sickle-cell) analysis, first determine p and q. With the frequencies of all the genotypes, one can add

0.756 and 0.242/2 to provide p ($= 0.877$); q will be
$1 - 0.877$ or 0.123

The equilibrium values will be as follows:

Frequency of AA $= p^2$ $= (0.877)^2 = 0.7691$ or 76.91%

Frequency of AS $= 2pq$ $= 2(0.877)(0.123) = 0.2157$ or 21.57%

Frequency of SS $= q^2$ $= (0.123)^2 = 0.0151$ or 1.51%

Comparing these equilibrium values with the observed values suggests that the observed values may be drawn from a population that is not in equilibrium. Notice that there are more heterozygotes than predicted, and fewer SS types in the population. Because data are given in percentages, χ^2 values cannot be computed.

22-3. Given that the recessive allele *a* is present in the homozygous state (q^2) at a frequency of 0.0001, the value of *q* is 0.01 and *p* = 0.99.

(a) *q* is 0.01

(b) *p* = 1 – *q* or 0.99

(c) $2pq$ = 2(0.01)(0.99) = 0.0198 (or about 1/50)

(d) $2pq \times 2pq$ = 0.0198 × 0.0198 = 0.000392 (or about 1/255)

22-4. The probability that the woman (with no family history of CF) is heterozygous is $2pq$ or 2(1/50)(49/50). The probability that the man is heterozygous is 2/3. The probability that a child with CF will be produced by two heterozygotes is 1/4. Therefore, the overall probability of the couple producing a CF child is 98/2500 × 2/3 × 1/4 = 0.00653, or about 1/153.

Chapter 22 Population and Evolutionary Genetics

Solutions to Problems and Discussion Questions

1. (a) Genetic variation can be assessed in a variety of ways, including responses to artificial selection and sequencing of nucleic acids and proteins.

(b) Different alleles will show typical segregation patterns and have similarities in nucleotide and amino acid sequences.

(c) By conducting assays of gene and/or genotypic frequencies over time and space, one can determine whether the genetic structure of a population is changing.

(d) If gene flow between populations becomes sufficiently reduced, divergence may have reached a point where the populations are reproductively isolated. Under this condition, they are usually considered different species.

(e) Various molecular clocks can be used to estimate the time of divergence of two groups of organisms. Such clocks are based on amino acid and/or nucleotide differences and are often validated by comparison with the fossil record.

2. Because of degeneracy in the code, there are some nucleotide substitutions, especially in the third base, that do not change amino acids. In addition, if there is no change in the overall charge of the protein, it is likely that electrophoresis will not separate the variants. If a positively charged amino acid is replaced by an amino acid of like charge, then the overall charge on the protein is unchanged. The same may be said for other negatively charged and neutral amino acid substitutions.

3. (a) Missense mutations cause amino acid changes.

(b) Horizontal transfer refers to the process of passing genetic information from one organism to another without producing offspring. In bacteria, plasmid transfer is an example of horizontal transfer.

(c) The fact that none of the isolates shared identical nucleotide changes indicates that there is little genetic exchange among different strains. Each alteration is unique, most likely originating in an ancestral strain and maintained in descendents of that strain only.

4. The classification of organisms into different species is based on evidence (morphological, genetic, ecological, etc.) that they are reproductively isolated. That is, there must be evidence that gene flow does not occur among the groups being called different species. Classifications above the species level (genus, family, etc.) are not based on such empirical data. Indeed, classification above the species level is somewhat arbitrary and based on traditions that extend far beyond DNA sequence information. In addition, recall that DNA sequence divergence is not always directly proportional to morphological, behavioral, or ecological divergence. Although the genus classifications provided in this problem seem to be invalid, other factors, well beyond simple DNA sequence comparison, must be considered in classification practices. As more information is gained on the meaning of DNA sequence differences in comparison to morphological factors, many phylogenetic relationships will be reconsidered, and it is possible that adjustments will be needed in some classification schemes.

5. There are many sections of DNA in a eukaryotic genome that are not reflected in a protein product. Indeed, there are many sections of DNA that are not even transcribed and/or have no apparent physiological role. Such regions are more likely to tolerate nucleotide changes compared with those regions with a necessary physiological impact. Introns, for example, show sequence variation, which is not reflected in a protein product. Exons, on the other hand, code for products that are usually involved in production of a phenotype and, as such, are subject to selection.

6. Understanding the Hardy–Weinberg equilibrium allows us to state that if a population is in equilibrium, the genotypic frequencies will not shift from one generation to the next unless there are factors such as selection or migration that alter gene frequencies. Because none of these factors is stated in the problem, we need only to determine whether the initial population is in equilibrium. Calculate p and q, then apply the equation $p^2 + 2pq + q^2$ to determine genotypic frequencies in the next generation.

$$p = \text{frequency of A}$$
$$= 0.2 + 0.3$$
$$= 0.5$$
$$q = 1 - p = 0.5$$

$$\text{Frequency of } AA = p^2$$
$$= (0.5)^2$$
$$= 0.25 \text{ or } 25\%$$

$$\text{Frequency of } Aa = 2pq$$
$$= 2(0.5)(0.5)$$
$$= 0.5 \text{ or } 50\%$$

Chapter 22 Population and Evolutionary Genetics

Frequency of $aa = q^2$
$$= (0.5)^2$$
$$= 0.25 \text{ or } 25\%$$

The initial population was not in equilibrium; however, after one generation of mating under the Hardy–Weinberg conditions, the population is in equilibrium and will continue to be so (and not change) until one or more of the Hardy–Weinberg conditions is not met. Note that *equilibrium* does not necessarily mean p and q equal 0.5.

7. For each of these values, one merely takes the square root to determine q, then computes p, then "plugs" the values into the $2pq$ expression.

(a) $q = 0.08$; $\quad 2pq = 2(0.92)(0.08)$
$$= 0.1472 \text{ or } 14.72\%$$

(b) $q = 0.009$; $\quad 2pq = 2(0.991)(0.009)$
$$= 0.01784 \text{ or } 1.78\%$$

(c) $q = 0.3$; $\quad 2pq = 2(0.7)(0.3)$
$$= 0.42 \text{ or } 42\%$$

(d) $q = 0.1$; $\quad 2pq = 2(0.9)(0.1)$
$$= 0.18 \text{ or } 18\%$$

(e) $q = 0.316$; $\quad 2pq = 2(0.684)(0.316)$
$$= 0.4323 \text{ or } 43.23\%$$

(Depending how one rounds off the decimals, slightly different answers will occur.)

8. In order for the Hardy–Weinberg equations to apply, the population must be in Hardy–Weinberg equilibrium.

9. Assuming that the population is in Hardy–Weinberg equilibrium, if one has the frequency of individuals with the dominant phenotype, the remainder have the recessive phenotype (q^2). With q^2, one can calculate q and from this value, one can arrive at p. Applying the expression $p^2 + 2pq + q^2$ will allow a solution to the question.

10. Given that $q^2 = 0.04$, then $q = 0.2$, $2pq = 0.32$, and $p^2 = 0.64$. Of those not expressing the trait, only a mating between heterozygotes can produce an offspring that expresses the trait, and then only at a frequency of 1/4. The different types of matings possible (those without the trait) in the population, with their frequencies, follow:

$AA \times AA = 0.64 \times 0.64 = 0.4096$
$AA \times Aa = 0.64 \times 0.32 = 0.2048$
$Aa \times AA = 0.64 \times 0.32 = 0.2048$

$Aa \times Aa = 0.32 \times 0.32 = 0.1024$
$Aa \times Aa = 0.32 \times 0.32 = 0.1024$

Notice that of the matings of the individuals who do not express the trait, only the last two (about 20 percent) are capable of producing offspring with the trait. Therefore, one would arrive at a final likelihood of 1/4 × 20 percent or 5 percent of the offspring with the trait.

11. The following formula calculates the frequency of an allele in the next generation for any selection scenario, given the frequencies of a and A in this generation and the fitness of all three genotypes;

$$q_{g+1} = [w_{Aa}p_gq_g + w_{aa}q_g^2]/[w_{AA}p_g^2 + w_{Aa}2p_gq_g + w_{aa}q_g^2]$$

where q_{g+1} is the frequency of the a allele in the next generation, q_g is the frequency of the a allele in this generation, p_g is the frequency of the A allele in this generation, and each "w" represents the fitness of its respective genotype.

(a) $q_{g+1} = [0.9(0.7)(0.3) + 0.8(0.3)^2]/[1(0.7)^2$
$$+ 0.9(2)(0.7)(0.3) + 0.8(.3)^2]$$

$q_{g+1} = 0.278$ $\quad p_{g+1} = 0.722$

(b) $q_{g+1} = 0.289$ $\quad p_{g+1} = 0.711$

(c) $q_{g+1} = 0.298$ $\quad p_{g+1} = 0.702$

(d) $q_{g+1} = 0.319$ $\quad p_{g+1} = 0.681$

12. The general equation for responding to this question is

$$q_n = q_o /(1 + nq_o)$$

where n = the number of generations, q_o = the initial gene frequency, and q_n = the new gene frequency.

(a) $n = 1$

$q_n = q_o/(1 + nq_o)$
$q_n = 0.5/[1 + (1 \times 0.5)]$
$q_n = 0.33$ $\quad p_n = 0.67$

(b) $n = 5$

$q_n = q_o/(1 + nq_o)$
$q_n = 0.5/[1 + (5 \times 0.5)]$
$q_n = 0.143$ $\quad p_n = 0.857$

(c) $n = 10$

$q_n = q_o/(1 + nq_o)$
$q_n = 0.5/[1 + (10 \times 0.5)]$
$q_n = 0.083$ $\quad p_n = 0.917$

204

(d) $n = 25$

$q_n = q_0/(1 + nq_0)$
$q_n = 0.5/[1 + (25 \times 0.5)]$
$q_n = 0.037 \qquad p_n = 0.963$

(e) $n = 100$

$q_n = q_0/(1 + nq_0)$
$q_n = 0.5/[1 + (100 \times 0.5)]$
$q_n = 0.0098 \qquad p_n = 0.9902$

(f) n = 1000

$q_n = q_0/(1 + nq_0)$
$q_n = 0.5/[1 + (1000 \times 0.5)]$
$q_n = 0.00099 \qquad p_n = 0.99901$

13. Because a dominant lethal gene is highly selected against, it is unlikely that it will exist at too high a frequency, if at all. However, if the gene shows incomplete penetrance or late age of onset (after reproductive age), it may remain in a population.

14. What one must do is predict the probability of one of the grandparents being heterozygous in this problem. Given the frequency of the disorder in the population as 1 in 10,000 individuals (0.0001), then $q^2 = 0.0001$, and $q = 0.01$. The frequency of heterozygosity is $2pq$, or approximately 0.02, as also stated in the problem. The probability for one of the grandparents to be heterozygous would therefore be $0.02 + 0.02$ or 0.04 or 1/25. (Note: If one considers the probability of both parents being carriers, 0.02×0.02, the answer differs slightly.) If one of the grandparents is a carrier, then the probability of the offspring from a first-cousin mating being homozygous for the recessive gene is 1/16. Multiplying the two probabilities together gives $1/16 \times 1/25 = 1/400$.

Following the same analysis for the second-cousin mating gives $1/64 \times 1/25 = 1/1600$. Notice that the population at large has a frequency of homozygotes of 1/10,000; therefore, one can easily see how inbreeding increases the likelihood of homozygosity.

15. The frequency of an allele is determined by a number of factors, including the fitness it confers, mutation rate, and input from migration. There is no tendency for a gene to reach any artificial frequency such as 0.5. In fact, you have seen that rare alleles tend to remain rare even when they are dominant—

unless there is very strong selection for the allele. The distribution of a gene among individuals is determined by mating (population size, inbreeding, etc.) and environmental factors (selection, etc.). A population is in Hardy–Weinberg equilibrium when the distribution of genotypes occurs at or around the $p^2 + 2pq + q^2 = 1$ expression. Equilibrium does not mean 25 percent *AA*, 50 percent *Aa*, and 25 percent *aa*. This confusion often stems from the 1:2:1 (or 3:1) ratio seen in Mendelian crosses.

16. During speciation, individuals or groups of potentially interbreeding organisms become genetically distinct from other members of the species. Members of different populations with substantial genetic divergence are, at first, not reproductively isolated from each other, although gene flow may be restricted. The distinction between such groups is not absolute in that one group may blend with other groups of the species. Any process that favors changes in allele frequencies has the potential of generating substantial genetic differences among different populations.

Factors such as selection, migration, genetic drift, or even mutation may be important in generating significant genetic change. One would certainly include geographic isolation as a major barrier to gene flow and thus an important process in such formation.

Natural selection occurs when there is nonrandom elimination of individuals from a population. Because such selection is a strong force in changing allele frequencies, it should also be considered as a significant factor in subspecies formation.

17. Because three of the affected infants had affected parents, only two "new" alleles, from mutation, enter into the problem. The allele is dominant; therefore, each new case of achondroplasia arose from a single new mutation. There are 50,000 births; therefore, 100,000 gametes (genes) are involved. The frequency of mutation is therefore given as follows: 2/100,000 or 2×10^{-5}.

18. The approximate similarity of mutation rates among genes and lineages should provide more credible estimates of divergence times of species and allow for broader interpretations of sequence comparisons. It also provides for increased understanding of the mutational processes that govern evolution among mammalian genomes. For instance, if the rate of mutation is fairly constant among lineages or cells that have a more rapid turnover, it indicates that replication-related errors do not make a significant contribution to mutation rates.

19. (a) The gene is most likely recessive because all affected individuals have unaffected parents and the condition clearly runs in families. For the population, because $q^2 = 0.002$, $q = 0.045$, $p = 0.955$, and $2(pq) = 0.086$. For the community, because $q^2 = 0.005$, $q = 0.07$, $p = 0.93$, and $2(pq) = 0.13$.

(b) The "founder effect" is probably operating here. Relatively small, local populations that are relatively isolated in a reproductive sense tend to show differences in gene frequencies when compared with larger populations. In such small populations, homozygosity is increased as a gene has a higher probability of "meeting itself" due to inbreeding.

20. Reproductive isolating mechanisms are grouped into prezygotic and postzygotic and include the following:

- geographic or ecological
- seasonal or temporal
- behavioral
- mechanical
- physiological
- hybrid inviability or weakness
- developmental hybrid sterility
- segregational hybrid sterility
- F_2 breakdown

21. Reproductive isolating mechanisms are grouped into prezygotic and postzygotic. Prezygotic mechanisms are more efficient because they occur before resources are expended in the processes of mating.

22. (a) Because noncoding genomic regions are probably silent genetically, it is likely that they contribute little, if anything, to the phenotype. Selection acts on the phenotype; therefore, such noncoding regions are probably selectively neutral.

(b) These polymorphism data indicate that all the Lake Victoria area (lake and contributing rivers) cichlids are related by recent ancestry, whereas those from neighboring lakes are more distantly related. In addition, because Lake Victoria dried out about 14,000 years ago, it is likely that it was repopulated by a relatively small sample of cichlids.

23. In general, speciation involves the gradual accumulation of genetic changes to a point where reproductive isolation occurs. Depending on environmental or geographic conditions, genetic changes may occur slowly or rapidly. They can involve point mutations or chromosomal changes.

24. Somatic gene therapy, like any therapy, allows some individuals to live more normal lives than those not receiving therapy. As such, the ability of such individuals to contribute to the gene pool increases the likelihood that less fit alleles will enter and be maintained in the gene pool. This is a normal consequence of therapy, genetic or not, and in the face of disease control and prevention, societies have generally accepted this consequence. Germ-line therapy could, if successful, lead to limited, isolated, and infrequent removal of an allele from a gene lineage. However, given the present state of the science, its impact on the course of human evolution will be diluted and negated by a host of other factors that afflict humankind.

25. (a,b) The pattern of genetic distances through time indicates that from the present to about 25,000 years ago, modern humans and Cro-Magnons show an approximately constant number of differences. Conversely, there is an abrupt increase in genetic distance seen in comparing modern humans and Cro-Magnons with Neanderthals. The results indicate a clear discontinuity among modern humans, Cro-Magnons, and Neanderthals with respect to genetic variation in the mitochondrial DNAs sampled. Assuming that the sampling and analytical techniques used to generate the data are valid, it appears that Neanderthals made little, if any, genetic contributions to the Cro-Magnon or modern European gene pool. It could be argued that the absence of Neanderthal mtDNA lineages in living humans is a consequence of random drift or lineage extinction since the disappearance of Neanderthals. However, the examination of ancient Cro-Magnon mtDNA shows no evidence of a historical relationship and suggests that Neanderthals were not genetically related to the ancestors of modern humans.

Chapter 23: Conservation Genetics

Concept Areas	Corresponding Problems
Genetic Diversity	1, 11, 12, 14
Population Dynamics	3
Management of Threatened Species	1, 2, 5, 9, 10, 12, 13, 15, 16, 17, 19, 20, 22
Small Populations	1, 4, 6, 17
Methods of Study	7, 8, 12, 15, 18, 21

Structures and Processes Checklist – Significant concepts that deserve special attention are identified with a "∗".

(check topic when mastered – provide examples where appropriate – understand the context of each entry)

- ○ **Introduction**
  - ○ human population growth*
  - ○ threatened species
  - ○ 2010 Red List*
  - ○ 25 percent of mammals
  - ○ 13 percent of birds
  - ○ 42 percent of amphibians
  - ○ 33 percent of reef-forming coral
  - ○ 30 percent of conifers
  - ○ loss of genetic diversity*
  - ○ biodiversity*
  - ○ ecosystem collapse*
  - ○ conservation genetics
- ○ **Genetic Diversity Is the Goal***
  - ○ interspecific diversity*
  - ○ intraspecific diversity*
  - ○ loss of genetic diversity
  - ○ population fragmentation*

- ○ gene flow
- ○ methods of study*
- ○ PCR
- ○ short tandem repeats
- ○ STRs
- ○ microsatellites
- ○ **Population Size***
  - ○ effective population size*
  - ○ population bottleneck*
  - ○ founder effect*
- ○ **Small, Isolated Populations***
  - ○ genetic drift*
  - ○ inbreeding*
  - ○ inbreeding coefficient (*F*)
  - ○ inbreeding depression*
  - ○ genetic load*
  - ○ reduction in gene flow
  - ○ metapopulation*

Chapter 23 Conservation Genetics

- **Genetic Erosion Threatens***
  - genetic erosion
  - outbred populations*
  - single-pair populations*
- **Genetic Diversity***
  - *ex situ* conservation*

- captive breeding*
- rescue examples
- gene banks*
- core collection
- *in situ* conservation*
- population augmentation*

Chapter 23 Conservation Genetics

Answers to Now Solve This

23-1. Apply the formula: $N_e = 4(N_m N_f)/N_m + N_f = 6.9$

23-2. (a) Apply the formula that computes the effective population size as the harmonic mean of the numbers in each generation:

$$N_e = 1/(1/t)(1/N_1 + 1/N_2 + 1/N_3 \ldots)$$

Substituting the values: $N_e = 1/(1/4)(1/47 + 1/17 + 1/20 + 1/35)$

$$N_e = 25.21$$

(b) Apply the formula that computes the frequency of heterozygotes after t generations as a function of effective population size:

$$H_t = (1 - 1/2N_e)^t H_o$$

Substituting the values: $H_t = (1 - 1/2(25.21))^4 (0.55)$

$$H_t = 0.5073$$

(c) Apply the formula that relates the inbreeding coefficient to the frequency of heterozygotes in a population:

$$F = (2pq - H)/2pq$$

$$F = (0.55 - 0.5073)/0.55$$

$$F = 0.0776$$

23-3. (a) The probability of being a heterozygote is $2pq = 2(0.99)(0.01) = 0.0198$. Multiplying this value by 20 gives the probability of being heterozygous:

$$0.0198 \times 20 = 0.396$$

(b) To determine N_e use the following expression:

$$N_e/N = 0.42$$

$$N_e = 0.42 \times 50 = 21$$

$$H_t = (1 - 1/2N_e)^t H_o$$

$$= (1 - 1/42)^5 \times 0.0198$$

$$= 0.01755$$

$$H_t/H_o = 0.01755/0.0198 = 0.886$$

Therefore, there is a loss of approximately 11.4 percent heterozygosity after five generations.

Chapter 23 Conservation Genetics

Solutions to Problems and Discussion Questions

1. (a) Genetic diversity in a species can be determined in a number of ways that include both obvious visual and more cryptic molecular markers. Allozyme assessments and DNA fingerprinting using short tandem repeats or microsatellites provide indices of genetic diversity.

(b) Numerous examples from a variety of observations and experiments indicate that as genetic diversity decreases, chances of a population's long-term survival also decrease. Natural examples include the peppered moth (*Biston betularia*), lions, seals, woodpeckers, and others. Laboratory studies using *Drosophila melanogaster* indicate that a loss of genetic diversity reduces the ability of a population to adapt to changing environments. Such a loss of adaptability diminishes chances for long-term survival.

(c) Any population that is of relatively small size will have a limited number of effective breeders. Mathematically, this increases the degree of allelic fluctuation and in many cases leads to elimination of alleles. Numerous studies indicate that the degree of allelic loss is greater in small populations where genetic drift is most likely.

(d) Population augmentation provides a variety of opportunities to increase genetic diversity. An increase in genetic diversity is often a prerequisite for species survival.

(e) In addition to attempts to maintain the genetic health of species by the conservation methods mentioned above, often as a last resort, gene banks are established to preserve reproductive components such as sperm, ova, and embryos.

2. The frequency (rough estimate because of small sample size) of the lethal allele in the captive population ($q^2 = 5/169$ and $q = 0.172$) is approximately double that in the gene pool as a whole ($q = 0.09$). Applying the formula

$$q_n = q_o/(1 + nq_o)$$

one can estimate that it would take 10 generations to reduce the lethal gene's frequency to 0.063 in the captive population with no intervention (random mating assumed). Because condors produce very few eggs per year, a more proactive approach seems justified.

(a) First, if detailed records are kept of the breeding partners of the captive birds, then knowledge of heterozygotes should be available. Breeding programs could be established to restrict matings between those carrying the lethal gene. Such "kinship management " is often used in captive populations. If kinship records are not available, it is often possible to establish kinship using genetic markers such as DNA microsatellite polymorphisms. Using such markers, one can often identify mating partners and link them to their offspring.

(b) By coupling knowledge of mating partners with the likelihood of producing a lethal genetic combination, selective matings can often be used to minimize the influence of a deleterious allele. In addition, such markers can be used to establish matings that optimize genetic mixing, thus reducing inbreeding depression.

3. Notice (in the text) that the probability of fixation through drift is the same as a gene's initial frequency. In this problem, the probability of A being fixed (and therefore a lost) is 0.75. The probability of B being fixed (and b being lost) is 0.8, and the probability of C being fixed (and c being lost) is 0.95. Therefore, the probability that all the recessive alleles will be lost through genetic drift is

$$0.75 \times 0.80 \times 0.95 = 0.57$$

4. Both genetic drift and inbreeding tend to drive populations toward homozygosity. Genetic drift is more common when the effective breeding size of the population is low. When this condition prevails, inbreeding is also much more likely. They are different in that inbreeding can occur when certain population structures or behaviors favor matings between relatives, regardless of the effective size of the population. Inbreeding tends to increase the frequency of both homozygous classes at the expense of the heterozygotes. Genetic drift can lead to fixation of one allele or the other, thus producing a single homozygous class.

5. There are a number of dangers inherent in the management of such a small herd of endangered rhinos. Because of the small breeding pool, inbreeding depression is likely to lead to less fit individuals over time. To combat this problem, genetic markers (such as microsatellites) can be used to assess the general degree of relatedness and heterozygosity of each of the 16 rhinos. From such information, appropriate matings can be facilitated that would reduce inbreeding depression. However, additional efforts may be needed in this extreme case. It is possible to develop exchange programs whereby animals from other herds provide semen (either naturally or artificially), thereby reducing inbreeding. This practice can be successful if females are receptive and if no deleterious alleles are brought into the population (outbreeding depression).

Population augmentation, whereby individuals are transplanted into a declining population, can be used to increase numbers and genetic diversity. However, as stated above, outbreeding depression may accompany this practice. Sometimes drastic measures must be taken in extreme cases such as the black rhino. Dehorning is often practiced to remove the incentive for poaching and reduce lethal wounding from fighting. This practice is only useful in areas devoid of dangerous predators.

6. Inbreeding depression, over time, reduces the level of heterozygosity, usually a selectively advantageous quality of a species. When homozygosity increases (through loss of heterozygosity), deleterious alleles are likely to become more of a load on a population. Outbreeding depression occurs when there is a reduction in fitness of progeny from genetically diverse individuals. It is usually attributed to offspring being less well-adapted to the local environmental conditions of the parents. Even though forced outbreeding may be necessary to save a threatened species, when population numbers are low, it significantly and permanently changes the genetic makeup of the species.

7. Cloning of some highly threatened species may be the only way to save that species from extinction. However, the long-term disadvantages of cloning for this purpose are often considered self-defeating. With cloning, one "short-circuits " normal processes (meiosis, gametic union, etc.) necessary to maintain genetic variation. With a loss of genetic variation come difficulties with adaptation as environments change. It may be possible to identify certain conditions in which cloning would be useful to "save" a species; however, interbreeding provides benefits that allow a species to evolve. In addition, as members of a species become more uniform (through cloning), they are more likely to suffer more severe and widespread responses to disease and environmental stress.

8. Often, molecular assays of overall heterozygosity can indicate the degree of inbreeding and/or genetic drift. As inbreeding and genetic drift, for that matter, occur, the degree of heterozygosity decreases. An

allele that has its frequency dictated by inbreeding will not be uniquely influenced. That is, other alleles would be characterized by decreased heterozygosity as well. So, if the genome in general has a relatively high degree of heterozygosity, the gene is probably influenced by selection rather than inbreeding and/or genetic drift.

9. *Ex situ* conservation involves the removal of an organism from an original habitat to an artificially maintained habitat. *In situ* conservation is an attempt to preserve a species in its original habitat. Each confronts problems. Although it may be possible to maintain an organism in an artificial habitat, it is no longer subject to the same selective pressures as experienced in the wild. Thus, the population will change. Attempts to maintain original habitats for *in situ* conservation are often met with failure as factors beyond a conservationist's control may dominate (air pollution, encroachment, and other aspects of habitat deterioration).

10. Generally, threatened species are captured and bred in an artificial environment until sufficient population numbers are achieved to ensure species survival. Next, genetic management strategies are applied to breed individuals in such a way as to increase genetic heterozygosity as much as possible. If plants are involved, seed banks are often used to maintain and facilitate long-term survival.

11. Genetic diversity generally increases the likelihood of long-term survival of a species by providing multiple opportunities for adaptation to environmental change. The ability of an organism to exploit varied environments and withstand environmental modification is directly related to genetic diversity.

12. Allozymes are variants of a particular protein often detected by electrophoresis. Such variation may or may not impact the fitness of an individual. The greater the allozyme variation, the more genetically heterogeneous the individual. It is generally agreed that such genetic diversity is essential for long-term survival. All other factors being equal, allozyme variation is more likely to reflect physiological variation than RFLP variation because RFLPs regions are not necessarily found in protein-coding regions of the genome. RFLP analysis allows one to detect very small amounts of genetic diversity in a population and is unlikely to encounter an organism that is not in some way variable in terms of RFLP with respect to other organisms (within and among species).

13. The maximum genetic diversity of the population will be enhanced by using the largest possible number in the founding population and minimizing the number of generations in captivity. By keeping complete pedigree records, one can increase genetic variation by reducing inbreeding and exchanging breeding individuals among captive populations.

14. Data from *Antechinus* provide insight as to the significance of genetic diversity to the survival of a species. Because such mechanisms (i.e., sperm mixing) are in place, there must be considerable evolutionary rewards. In this case, maintaining diversity must offset the cost (if any) of evolving such a mechanism.

15. (a) Maintenance of heterozygosity in a population is dependent on a number of factors including degree of inbreeding, population size, and mutational input through migration and/or mutation. If a population is small and isolated, inbreeding and genetic drift are likely consequences. Both decrease heterozygosity. Coupled with lessened connections with neighboring populations, reduced heterozygosity is expected.

(b) Urbanization usually leads to fragmentation of natural populations as highways, strip malls, and housing developments disrupt the natural habitat and, as a consequence, the movements of organisms. Even though two populations may be relatively close to each other geographically, they may be genetically distant because of restricted movement. Restricted movement between and among such populations will foster genetic diversity.

(c) In general, restrictions to movements must be greatly reduced or eliminated. Safe corridors for passage over or under highways and through populated areas must be developed. Unless population augmentation is to be employed, native populations must be able to maintain sufficient genetic diversity through interbreeding in order to survive.

16. (a) Because prairie dogs are the main food source for black-footed ferrets, a reduction in prairie dogs would likely stress black-footed ferrets. Unless alternate food sources are available and utilized by the ferrets, their numbers would decline.

(b) Because a population survives a population bottleneck does not mean that the population is in a healthy state. Usually, bottlenecks reduce genetic variability upon which survival and adaptation depend. A second bottleneck, although perhaps not having immediate ramifications, would likely have a negative impact on the long-term survival of the species. One would expect additional reductions in genetic diversity.

(c) Because extinction of an organism is irreversible, one might consider the fate of the ferret as the highest priority. If the prairie dog population is reduced very slowly, the ferret population may succeed in finding alternative food sources, but this is doubtful. Because the ferret population is the most fragile of the three (ferret, prairie dog, cattle) and represents one of America's most endangered mammals, this case will test the strength of laws designed to protect such species. In some situations, compromise to the point of mutual agreement is not possible.

17. First, it will be necessary to determine whether the native habitat in the Asian steppes of the 1920s is suitable to any introduction. If the original range is supportive of reintroduction, care must be taken to introduce horses with the maximum genetic diversity possible. To do so, you might monitor RFLP patterns. Because the founder breeding group included a domestic mare, it may be desirable to select those for reintroduction that are least like the domestic mare genetically. It might be desirable to release reasonably sized breeding groups in separate locations within the range to enhance eventual genetic diversity.

18. DNA profiles indicate the degree of heterogeneity in DNA sequences and therefore the degree of genetic variation. Whereas non-coding DNA sequences represent the bulk of sequence diversity, such information can be helpful in determining gene flow, ancestry, and overall inter- and intra-population diversity. Because diversity *per se* appears to be essential for long-term species survival in natural environments, one would expect that the assessment of diversity by any tool will be a useful predictor.

19. From a physiological standpoint, cryogenic preservation in liquid nitrogen can allow 100 years or more of seed storage for some species; however, such elaborate storage can be offered to only a small fraction of the world's seeds. Thus, seeds of most species undergo storage loss, which decreases genetic diversity. Seeds of tropical plants are somewhat intolerant to cold storage and must be regenerated frequently, a practice that is prone to a loss of genetic diversity arising from genetic drift. Only a finite number of seeds can be used in each regeneration procedure, and the restriction of sample size (often fewer than 100 plants) reduces genetic diversity. To somewhat counteract this problem, plants are grown under optimum conditions to reduce selection. Another problem associated with preserved seeds is the accumulation of deleterious mutations both as a result of seed storage and regeneration. Some studies indicate increased frequencies of chromosomal and mtDNA lesions, chlorophyll deficiency mutations, and decreased DNA polymerase activity associated with long-term seed storage.

20. A census of population size and range would be needed to establish levels of habitat exploitation and probable number of effective breeding pairs. From this information, an estimation of long-term habitat support can be provided along with the probability of genetic drift eroding genetic variability. Effective breeder estimates will also provide a method for estimating inbreeding depression. It would be helpful to conduct surveys on a season-to-season and year-to-year basis to decrease the possibility of sampling in an atypical season or year. It would be important to determine the age and stage-specific structure of the endangered population. Few young or juveniles might indicate that reproductive capacities are in decline. It would be important to determine the general level of biodiversity and carrying capacity of the habitat as well as the genetic diversity of the species in question. Nuclear, mitochondrial, and chloroplast DNA profiles can be used to assess intrapopulation and interpopulation variation as well as to aid in determining migration and breeding patterns.

21. The longest bottleneck-to-present interval occurred with cheetahs, and one would expect cheetahs to show the highest degree of microsatellite polymorphism. The shortest bottleneck-to-present interval occurred with the Gir Forest lions, so it would be expected to have the least polymorphism. Data from Driscoll et al. (2002 *Genome Research* 12:414–423) include the following estimates of

microsatellite polymorphism in the three feline groups mentioned above: cheetahs (84.1%), pumas (42.9%), and Gir Forest lions (19.3%). The following graph would incorporate the expected relationship between bottlenecks and microsatellite variation.

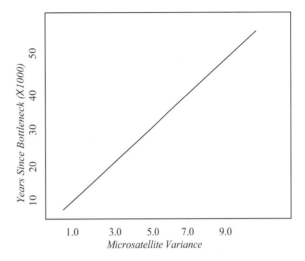

22. Although flagship species (often large mammals) may make it possible to gather considerable public support and funding, they may reduce support for species that may have a greater impact on a community of species. Primary producers (plants) are a necessary component of a diverse and supportive habitat. If one focuses on a flagship species within an area, it is possible that other areas will suffer more dramatically because foundational species are lost. Using umbrella species to protect a large geographic area in hopes of protecting other species in that area is a reasonable approach. However, the size of an area is not necessarily a primary factor in determining species success. Diversity and productivity of a habitat are major contributors to species success. Because land is at a premium, it may be wiser in the long run to select umbrella species in diverse and productive habitats rather than on the basis of land size.

By selecting sets of species that show considerable biodiversity, one increases the likelihood of protecting a sufficiently rich habitat to support many species. Such habitats are often of considerable economic value, thereby limiting their availability.